ATI TEAS SIMPLIFIED
STUDY GUIDE

Summary

INTRODUCTION

THE FIRST STEP IS YOU

"Success is a journey, not a destination."

It begins with a single step, a commitment to your goals, and the determination to overcome every obstacle in your way. As you embark on this path, it's essential to understand that success is not a linear progression but a series of peaks and valleys. Each challenge you encounter is an opportunity for growth, each setback a lesson in resilience.

The first step on this journey is setting a clear vision of what success looks like for you. Whether it's achieving top marks in your exams, gaining admission to your dream college, or excelling in a particular subject, having a defined goal gives you a target to aim for. This vision should be vivid and compelling, something that motivates you to push through the tough times.

Once you have your vision, break it down into smaller, manageable goals. These milestones will serve as checkpoints along your journey, allowing you to measure your progress and make necessary adjustments. Each small victory will build your confidence and keep you motivated.

Building Confidence and Competence

Confidence and competence are two sides of the same coin. Building one often leads to the development of the other. Competence comes from practice and mastery of a subject, while confidence arises from the recognition of this competence.

To build competence, immerse yourself in your studies. Engage with the material actively through reading, writing, and discussion. Seek to understand concepts deeply rather than memorizing facts. Use a variety of resources – books, online courses, study groups – to gain different perspectives.

Confidence, on the other hand, can be cultivated through positive self-talk and visualization techniques. Imagine yourself succeeding, achieving your goals, and overcoming obstacles. Celebrate your achievements, no matter how small, and remind yourself of your progress regularly. Combining these strategies, you'll find that as your competence grows, so does your confidence. And with confidence, you'll be more willing to take on challenges and stretch your capabilities further.

Personalized Study Strategies

Every student is unique, and so are their study needs. Personalized study strategies are crucial for maximizing your learning potential. The first step in developing a personalized study plan is understanding your learning style. Are you a visual learner who benefits from diagrams and videos, an auditory learner who retains information better through listening, or a kinesthetic learner who needs hands-on activities?

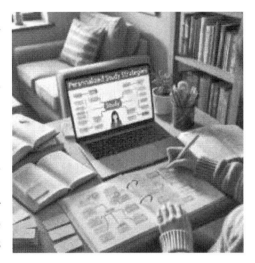

Once you know your learning style, tailor your study methods to suit it. Visual learners might create mind maps or flashcards, while auditory learners could benefit from recording their notes and listening to them. Kinesthetic learners might use physical objects to represent concepts or engage in activities that require movement.

Time management is another critical aspect of personalized study strategies. Create a study schedule that allocates time for each subject based on its difficulty and your comfort level with the material. Be sure to include breaks to avoid burnout and maintain productivity.

Overcoming Test Anxiety

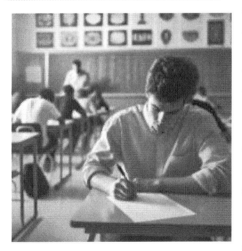

Test anxiety is a common issue that can hinder performance despite thorough preparation. The key to overcoming test anxiety lies in preparation and mindset. Start by familiarizing yourself with the test format and practicing under similar conditions. This reduces the fear of the unknown and builds confidence.

Developing relaxation techniques such as deep breathing, visualization, and progressive muscle relaxation can help manage anxiety. Practice these techniques regularly so that they become second nature during the test.

Positive self-talk is also essential. Replace negative thoughts like "I can't do this" with affirmations such as "I am well-prepared and capable." Visualization techniques can also be helpful; imagine yourself calmly and confidently taking the test and achieving your desired score.

Additionally, maintaining a healthy lifestyle can significantly impact your anxiety levels. Regular exercise, a balanced diet, and adequate sleep are all crucial for optimal brain function and stress management.

Insider Tips from Top Scorers

Learning from those who have succeeded before you can provide invaluable insights. Top scorers often attribute their success to specific strategies and habits. One common tip is to start studying early and consistently. Cramming might work for some, but long-term retention and understanding come from regular review.

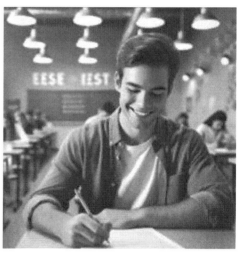

Top scorers also emphasize the importance of practice tests. These not only familiarize you with the test format but also help identify areas of weakness. Reviewing your mistakes and understanding why you got a question wrong is crucial for improvement.

Another tip is to create a distraction-free study environment. This means finding a quiet place where you can focus entirely on your studies. Some top scorers even suggest studying in different locations to keep the mind stimulated and avoid monotony.

Setting Realistic and Achievable Goals

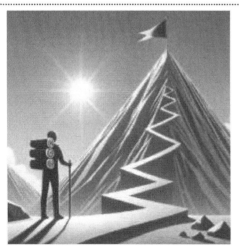

Goal setting is a powerful tool for success, but it's essential to set goals that are both realistic and achievable. Unrealistic goals can lead to frustration and burnout, while achievable goals provide a sense of accomplishment and motivation.

Start by setting **SMART goals – Specific, Measurable, Achievable, Relevant, and Time-bound**. For example, instead of setting a vague goal like "study more," set a specific goal such as "study for two hours every day after school."

Break down your long-term goals into smaller, manageable tasks. This not only makes the goal seem less daunting but also allows you to track your progress more effectively. Each completed task brings you one step closer to your ultimate goal, boosting your confidence and motivation.

Remember to celebrate your achievements, no matter how small. This positive reinforcement helps maintain your motivation and commitment to your goals.

In conclusion, embarking on your path to success requires a clear vision, confidence, personalized study strategies, effective management of test anxiety, insights from top scorers, and realistic goal setting. By integrating these elements into your routine, you'll be well-equipped to navigate the journey to success.

WHAT IS THE ATI TEAS?

The **ATI TEAS (Test of Essential Academic Skills)** exam is a pivotal stepping stone for many aspiring healthcare professionals. Designed to assess the fundamental academic skills required for a career in healthcare, this test is crucial for entry into nursing and allied health programs. Understanding its structure and components is the first step towards conquering this challenge.

The TEAS exam covers four main areas: Reading, Mathematics, Science, and English and Language Usage. Each section evaluates specific skills essential for academic and professional success in healthcare. The Reading section tests comprehension and interpretation abilities. Mathematics assesses basic arithmetic, algebra, and data interpretation skills. Science covers human anatomy, life and physical sciences, and scientific reasoning. Lastly, the English and Language Usage section focuses on grammar, punctuation, and language conventions.

What to Expect on Test Day?

Test day can be nerve-wracking, but knowing what to expect can help alleviate some of the anxiety. The first thing to note is the importance of arriving early. Most testing centers recommend arriving at least 30 minutes before the scheduled start time. This allows ample time for check-in procedures, which typically include verifying your identity and securing personal belongings. Ensuring you have a valid ID, your test registration confirmation, and any other required documents can streamline the process and reduce stress.

Upon arrival, you'll be directed to a waiting area until the exam begins. This area is often filled with other test-takers, and the atmosphere can be a mix of nervous energy and focused anticipation. It's crucial to stay calm and composed during this time. Many find it helpful to engage in light conversation or practice deep breathing exercises to manage any pre-test jitters. Visualizing success and recalling your preparation can also boost your confidence.

The TEAS test is **a computer-based exam**, so familiarizing yourself with the testing software beforehand can be advantageous. The test is timed, with a total duration of **209 minutes**. Each section has a specific time limit: **Reading (64 minutes), Mathematics (54 minutes), Science (63 minutes),** and **English and Language Usage (28 minutes).** It's important to pace yourself to ensure you have enough time to answer all questions within each section.

Once the exam begins, you'll be led to your workstation equipped with a computer and necessary materials. The workstation is usually a small cubicle to minimize distractions, providing a quiet and focused environment. You'll be given instructions on how to navigate the testing software, including how to answer questions, review answers, and keep track of time.

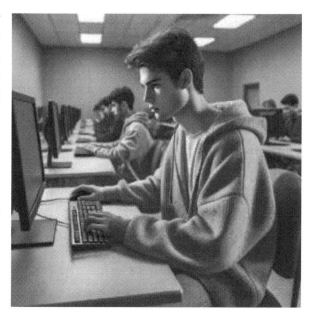

Before the actual test starts, there may be a short tutorial on the test interface. This is a good opportunity to familiarize yourself with the layout and functionality of the system, ensuring you know how to flag questions for review or skip and return to difficult ones.

The testing room is typically monitored by proctors who ensure the integrity of the exam and are available to address any technical issues that may arise. However, they will not answer any content-related questions. It's important to adhere to all testing center rules, such as not bringing unauthorized items into the exam room and maintaining a quiet environment.

During the test, it's essential to pace yourself. Keep an eye on the clock, but don't let it distract you. Most exams are divided into sections with specific time limits, so manage your time wisely to ensure you complete each section. If you encounter a difficult question, it's often best to move on and return to it later if time permits.

By understanding what to expect on test day and being well-prepared, you can reduce anxiety and increase your chances of performing at your best.

Essential Strategies for Test Success

Success on the TEAS exam hinges on a combination of preparation and strategy. Here are some essential strategies to maximize your performance:

Develop a Study Plan

Create a comprehensive study schedule that covers all four sections of the test. Allocate more time to areas where you feel less confident.

Utilize Practice Tests

Taking practice tests under timed conditions helps you get accustomed to the format and pacing of the exam. Analyze your performance to identify strengths and weaknesses.

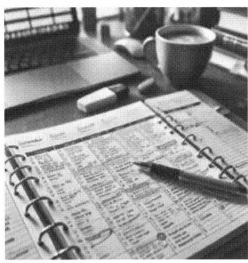

Focus on Weak Areas

Use your practice test results to guide your study sessions. Spend extra time reviewing concepts and practicing questions in areas where you scored lower.

Join Study Groups

Collaborating with peers can provide new insights and different perspectives on challenging topics. Study groups can also keep you motivated and accountable.

Seek Resources

Utilize study guides, online courses, and other resources tailored to the TEAS exam. These can provide structured content review and additional practice questions.

Maintain a Healthy Lifestyle

Proper nutrition, exercise, and adequate sleep are essential for optimal brain function. Ensure you're physically and mentally prepared for the test.

Understanding the Different Question Types

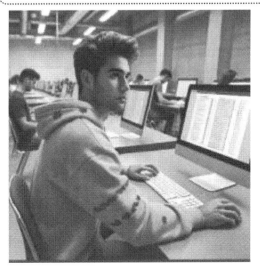

The TEAS exam includes a variety of question types, each designed to assess different skills and knowledge areas. Familiarizing yourself with these question types can improve your test-taking efficiency and accuracy.

Multiple-Choice Questions

These are the most common type of questions on the TEAS exam. Each question presents a statement or question followed by four answer choices. Your task is to select the best answer. Practice process-of-elimination techniques to narrow down your choices and improve your chances of selecting the correct answer.

Multiple-Select Questions

In these questions, you'll be required to select all correct answers from a list of options. There may be more than one correct answer, and you'll need to identify all of them to receive full credit. This question type requires careful reading and comprehensive understanding of the topic.

Fill-in-the-Blank Questions

These questions require you to type the correct answer into a blank space. They often test specific knowledge, such as mathematical calculations or vocabulary. Practice recalling information quickly and accurately to excel in these questions.

Hot Spot Questions

Hot spot questions involve identifying a specific area on an image or diagram. You'll click on the area that best answers the question. These questions are commonly found in the Science section and may involve labeling anatomical structures or identifying parts of a graph.

Ordered Response Questions

These questions require you to arrange a set of items in a specific order. They test your ability to understand sequences and processes. Practice ordering steps logically and reviewing processes, especially in scientific and mathematical contexts.

Mastering Time Management Techniques

Time management is crucial for success on the TEAS exam. With a limited amount of time for each section, it's essential to pace yourself and ensure you have enough time to answer all questions. Here are some techniques to help you manage your time effectively:

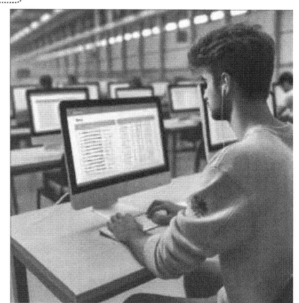

Prioritize Questions

Start by quickly scanning through the questions in each section. Answer the ones you find easiest first. This ensures you secure as many points as possible before tackling more challenging questions.

Use the Process of Elimination

For difficult multiple-choice questions, eliminate obviously incorrect answers first. This increases your chances of selecting the correct answer from the remaining options.

Keep an Eye on the Clock

Regularly check the time remaining in each section. If you find yourself spending too much time on a single question, make a note of it and move on. Return to it later if you have time left.

Practice Pacing

Use practice tests to develop a sense of timing for each section. Aim to complete each section slightly ahead of time to allow for review and revision of your answers.

Stay Calm and Focused

Maintain a steady pace and avoid rushing. Stay calm and focused, and don't let difficult questions shake your confidence. Deep breathing and positive self-talk can help maintain your composure.

Insights from Practice Tests

Practice tests are one of the most effective tools for preparing for the TEAS exam. They simulate the actual test environment, allowing you to become familiar with the format and timing. Here are some insights on how to use practice tests effectively:

- **Simulate Test Conditions**

  Take practice tests in a quiet environment, free from distractions. Time yourself to replicate the actual test conditions. This helps build stamina and concentration.

- **Review Your Answers**

  After completing a practice test, thoroughly review your answers. Identify the questions you got wrong and understand why. This helps pinpoint areas for improvement.

- **Track Your Progress**

  Keep a record of your practice test scores and monitor your progress over time. This allows you to see how your performance improves and which areas still need attention.

- **Analyze Patterns**

  Look for patterns in your mistakes. Are there certain types of questions you consistently get wrong? Are there specific topics you struggle with? Use this analysis to focus your study efforts.

- **Adjust Your Study Plan**

  Based on your practice test results, adjust your study plan. Spend more time on weak areas and continue to reinforce your strengths. Regularly updating your study plan ensures you remain focused and efficient.

- **Build Confidence**

  Regular practice tests help build confidence and reduce test anxiety. The more familiar you become with the test format and question types, the more comfortable you'll feel on test day.

In conclusion, preparing for the ATI TEAS exam requires a comprehensive approach that includes understanding the test structure, developing effective study strategies, mastering different question types, managing your time efficiently, and leveraging insights from practice tests. By integrating these elements into your preparation, you'll be well-equipped to achieve success on the TEAS exam and take a significant step towards your career in healthcare.

UNLOCKING THE FULL POTENTIAL OF THIS GUIDE

This guide is more than just a collection of study tips and practice questions; it's a comprehensive roadmap tailored to lead you through every step of your preparation journey. By leveraging the strategies and insights provided here, you will not only enhance your understanding of the material but also develop the confidence and skills needed to excel on test day.

This guide is structured to provide you with a holistic approach to studying, incorporating various methods and tools to cater to different learning styles. From creating a personalized study schedule to utilizing interactive study tools, every aspect is covered to ensure you are thoroughly prepared. Embrace this guide as your companion in your TEAS preparation, and let it guide you to success.

Navigating Your Study Journey

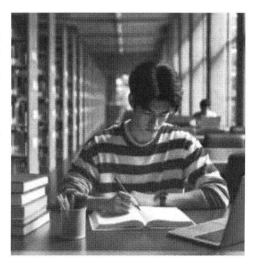

Embarking on your study journey for the ATI TEAS exam can feel overwhelming, but with a clear plan and the right mindset, it can be a rewarding experience. The key is to approach your studies systematically, breaking down the material into manageable chunks and setting achievable goals.

Start by familiarizing yourself with the structure of the TEAS exam. Knowing what to expect in each section—Reading, Mathematics, Science, and English and Language Usage—will help you identify areas where you need to focus your efforts. Create an overview of the topics covered in each section and assess your current knowledge and skills in relation to these topics.

Setting the Stage

Begin your study journey by setting up a dedicated study space that is free from distractions. A well-organized, quiet environment can significantly enhance your concentration and productivity. Equip your study space with all the necessary materials, such as textbooks, notebooks, highlighters, and a reliable computer or tablet.

Next, set clear, specific goals for what you want to achieve in each study session. Whether it's mastering a particular concept in algebra or improving your reading comprehension skills, having a defined objective will keep you focused and motivated. Use a planner or digital calendar to schedule your study sessions, ensuring you allocate enough time for each subject area.

Breaking Down the Material

To avoid feeling overwhelmed, break down the material into smaller, more manageable segments. This approach, known as chunking, allows you to focus on one topic at a time, making it easier to absorb and retain information. For instance, instead of trying to study all of human anatomy in one sitting, break it down into sections such as the skeletal system, muscular system, and cardiovascular system.

Incorporate a variety of study methods to keep your learning engaging and effective. Mix up reading, writing, and interactive activities like quizzes and flashcards. This not only prevents monotony but also caters to different aspects of memory retention.

Creating a Customized Study Schedule

A customized study schedule is crucial for efficient and effective preparation. It helps you stay organized, track your progress, and ensure you cover all necessary material before test day. Here's how to create a study schedule tailored to your needs.

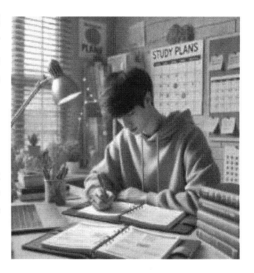

Assess Your Starting Point

Before you create your schedule, assess your current knowledge level. Take a diagnostic test to identify your strengths and weaknesses. This will give you a clear idea of which areas require more focus and time.

Set Realistic Goals

Setting realistic and achievable goals is essential. Break down your overall goal into smaller, weekly objectives. For example, you might aim to complete the mathematics section of your study guide by the end of the first week. Use the SMART criteria—Specific, Measurable, Achievable, Relevant, and Time-bound—to set your goals.

Plan Your Study Sessions

Once you have your goals, plan your study sessions accordingly. Allocate specific time blocks for each subject area, ensuring a balanced approach. For instance:
- Monday: 2 hours of Reading comprehension and analysis
- Tuesday: 1.5 hours of Algebra and 1.5 hours of Geometry
- Wednesday: 2 hours of Human Anatomy
- Thursday: 1 hour of Grammar and 1 hour of Vocabulary
- Friday: 2 hours of Chemistry and Biology
- Saturday: Practice test and review

Incorporate Breaks and Review Time

Don't forget to include short breaks in your schedule to avoid burnout. A 5-10 minute break after every hour of study can help maintain focus and productivity. Additionally, allocate time for review sessions at the end of each week to consolidate what you've learned and identify areas that may need further attention.

Utilizing All Available Resources for Optimal Learning

To maximize your learning potential, take advantage of all available resources. The more diverse your study materials, the better prepared you'll be for the exam.

Books and Study Guides

Invest in reputable TEAS study guides and textbooks. These resources provide comprehensive coverage of the exam content and often include practice questions and tests.

Online Courses and Tutorials

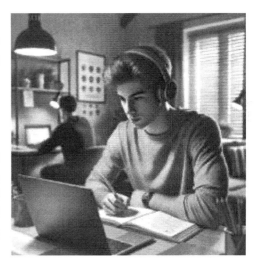

Online courses and tutorials offer flexibility and interactive learning opportunities. Websites like Khan Academy, Coursera, and Udemy offer courses that cover subjects tested on the TEAS exam. These platforms often include video lessons, quizzes, and discussion forums where you can ask questions and engage with other learners.

Practice Tests

Taking practice tests is one of the most effective ways to prepare for the TEAS exam. They help you familiarize yourself with the format, timing, and types of questions you'll encounter. Use official practice tests from ATI as well as other reputable sources to get a well-rounded practice experience.

Study Groups

Joining or forming a study group can provide additional support and motivation. Study groups allow you to discuss challenging topics, share resources, and quiz each other. They also offer a sense of accountability, helping you stay on track with your study schedule.

Interactive Study Tools and Techniques

Incorporating interactive study tools and techniques can make your study sessions more engaging and effective. Here are some tools and methods to consider:

Flashcards

Flashcards are a great way to reinforce key concepts and vocabulary. Use physical flashcards or digital apps like Anki or Quizlet, which allow you to create custom flashcards and access pre-made decks.

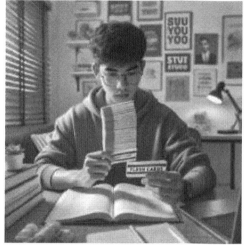

Mind Maps

Mind maps help you visualize connections between different concepts, making it easier to understand and remember complex information. Create mind maps for each subject area, linking key topics and subtopics. Tools like MindMeister or simple pen and paper can be used for this purpose.

Interactive Quizzes

Interactive quizzes are a fun way to test your knowledge and identify areas that need improvement. Websites like Kahoot and Quizizz offer customizable quizzes on a wide range of topics. Use these quizzes as a break from traditional study methods while still reinforcing your learning.

Study Apps

There are numerous study apps available that can aid in your TEAS preparation. Apps like Khan Academy, Brainscape, and TEAS Mastery provide interactive lessons, flashcards, and practice questions tailored to the TEAS exam.

Videos and Tutorials

Videos and tutorials can provide a different perspective on challenging topics. Platforms like YouTube, Khan Academy, and CrashCourse offer educational videos that explain complex concepts in an engaging and easily digestible format.

Monitoring and Tracking Your Progress

Regularly monitoring and tracking your progress is essential to ensure you're on the right path and to make necessary adjustments to your study plan.

Keeping a Study Journal

Maintaining a study journal can help you track your daily study activities, note important concepts, and reflect on your learning progress. Write down what you've studied each day, any difficulties you encountered, and how you overcame them. This not only helps with accountability but also provides a valuable resource for review.

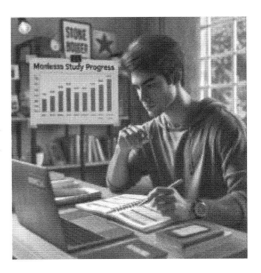

Using Progress Trackers

Progress trackers, such as charts or spreadsheets, can visually represent your study milestones and achievements. Update your tracker regularly to see how much you've accomplished and identify any gaps in your preparation.

Self-Assessments

Regular self-assessments, such as quizzes or practice tests, can help gauge your understanding of the material. Analyze your results to identify areas of improvement and adjust your study plan accordingly. Focus on your weak areas while continuing to reinforce your strengths.

Seeking Feedback

Don't hesitate to seek feedback from teachers, tutors, or study group members. They can provide valuable insights and suggestions to improve your study methods and understanding of the material. Constructive feedback can help you stay motivated and focused on your goals.

Staying Motivated

Staying motivated throughout your study journey is crucial for success. Set small rewards for yourself upon achieving study milestones, such as taking a break, enjoying a favorite snack, or spending time on a hobby. Remind yourself of your ultimate goal and the benefits of achieving it. Positive reinforcement and a clear sense of purpose can keep you motivated and committed to your study plan.

In conclusion, unlocking the full potential of this ATI TEAS Test guide requires a comprehensive approach that encompasses understanding the exam structure, creating a customized study schedule, utilizing various resources, incorporating interactive study tools, and continuously monitoring your progress. By following these strategies and maintaining a positive and proactive mindset, you will be well-prepared to excel on the TEAS exam and take a significant step towards your career in healthcare.

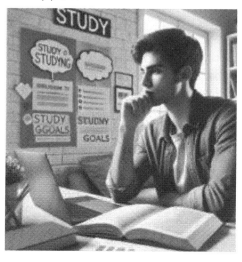

Detailed Content of the Book

The book is divided into four main units, each focusing on a critical area of the TEAS exam. Here's a closer look at what each unit contains and how to maximize its use:

Unit I - Conquering the World of Mathematics

This unit covers foundational mathematical concepts essential for the TEAS exam. Starting with basic arithmetic and advancing to more complex topics like algebra and data interpretation, this unit is designed to build your mathematical skills progressively.

- Foundations of Mathematical Mastery: Begin with the basics of arithmetic, whole numbers, and operations. Understanding these fundamentals is crucial as they form the building blocks for more advanced topics.
- Advancing Your Mathematical Skills: Dive into fractions, decimals, and percentages. These sections include practical examples and exercises to reinforce your understanding.
- Tackling Advanced Mathematical Challenges: Explore algebraic expressions, variables, equations, and inequalities. This section simplifies complex concepts, making them easier to grasp.
- Practical Applications of Mathematics: Learn how to

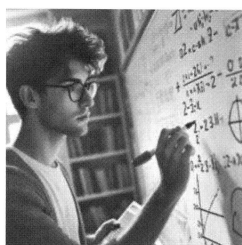

apply mathematical concepts in real-world scenarios, including measurement techniques, data visualization, and probability.

Unit II - Unveiling the Mysteries of Science

This unit delves into the scientific concepts tested on the TEAS exam, including human anatomy, physiology, life sciences, and physical sciences.

- Human Anatomy and Physiology Uncovered: Gain a comprehensive understanding of the human body, from cellular structures to organ systems. This section includes detailed explanations and diagrams to enhance your learning.
- Diving into Life Sciences: Study the fundamentals of DNA, genetics, cell division, ecosystems, and evolution. This section provides a holistic view of biological sciences.
- Exploring the Physical Sciences and Chemistry: Understand chemical reactions, the periodic table, and basic physics principles. This section demystifies complex scientific concepts with clear explanations and practical examples.
- Mastering Scientific Inquiry and Method: Learn about the scientific method, experimental design, and ethical considerations in research. This section helps you develop critical thinking skills essential for scientific inquiry.

Unit III - Excelling in Reading Comprehension

This unit focuses on enhancing your reading comprehension skills, crucial for success in the TEAS exam.

- Strategic Reading for Success: Develop strategies to identify main ideas, analyze the author's purpose, and draw inferences. This section includes practical tips and exercises to improve your reading efficiency.
- Enhancing Critical Reading Skills: Break down complex texts, navigate technical passages, and interpret visual information. This section helps you become a more analytical and critical reader.
- Practice Makes Perfect: Reading Comprehension: Engage with sample passages and practice questions. Detailed explanations help you understand the reasoning behind correct answers, improving your comprehension skills.

Unit IV - Mastering English and Language Usage

This unit covers essential grammar, vocabulary, and writing skills needed for the TEAS exam.

- Grammar and Syntax Essentials: Learn the rules of grammar, sentence structure, and punctuation. This section includes exercises to reinforce your understanding and correct common errors.
- Advanced Language Skills: Expand your vocabulary, use context clues, and understand idioms. This section helps you enhance your language skills and improve your writing style.
- Effective Communication Strategies: Develop persuasive writing skills, write for different purposes, and integrate feedback. This section includes practical writing prompts and exercises to improve your communication skills.

Practice Questions

In addition to the detailed content and strategies provided in each unit, this book includes a comprehensive set of practice questions. These questions are designed to simulate the types of questions you will encounter on the TEAS exam, providing you with the opportunity to apply what you have learned and assess your readiness. Each set of practice questions comes with detailed rationales to help you understand the reasoning behind the correct answers and learn from any mistakes.

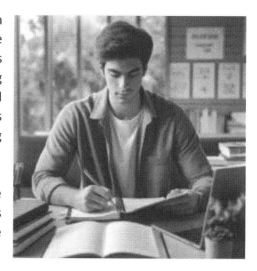

By systematically working through each unit and utilizing the interactive tools, practice questions, and additional resources provided, you can maximize your study efficiency and achieve success on the ATI TEAS exam.

FOUNDATIONS OF MATHEMATICAL MASTERY

Mathematics is often seen as the bedrock of logical reasoning, problem-solving, and analytical thinking. It is a universal language, a tool that allows us to quantify, measure, and understand the world around us. In this chapter, we embark on a journey to establish a robust foundation in mathematics, essential for excelling in the ATI TEAS exam. Our exploration will begin with the basic building blocks of arithmetic, gradually advancing towards more complex concepts.

The Language of Numbers

Understanding numbers is the first step toward mathematical proficiency. Numbers come in various forms and serve different purposes:

Type of Number	Definition	Examples
Natural Numbers	The simplest form of numbers, starting from 1 and increasing by increments of 1.	1, 2, 3, ...
Whole Numbers	Natural numbers along with 0.	0, 1, 2, 3, ...
Integers	Whole numbers including their negative counterparts.	-3, -2, -1, 0, 1, 2, 3, ...
Rational Numbers	Numbers that can be expressed as a fraction or ratio of two integers, where the denominator is not zero.	1/2, 2/3, 4/1, ...

These different types of numbers form the basis for more complex mathematical operations and concepts. Recognizing and working with each type effectively is crucial for problem-solving and higher-level mathematics.

Operations and Their Properties

Once familiar with numbers, the next step is mastering basic operations: addition, subtraction, multiplication, and division. Each operation has unique properties that simplify calculations and problem-solving.

Addition and Subtraction

Addition involves combining quantities, while subtraction involves finding the difference between quantities. These operations are governed by specific properties:

Property	Definition	Example
Commutative Property	The order of numbers does not change the sum.	$4 + 5 = 5 + 4$
Associative Property	The grouping of numbers does not change the sum.	$(2 + 3) + 4 = 2 + (3 + 4)$
Identity Property	Adding zero to a number does not change its value.	$7 + 0 = 7$
Inverse Property	The sum of a number and its negative is zero.	$6 + (-6) = 0$

Property	Definition	Example

Multiplication and Division

Multiplication and division are repeated addition and subtraction, respectively. These operations have their own sets of properties:

	Definition	Example
Commutative Property	The order of numbers does not change the product.	$3 \times 4 = 4 \times 3$
Associative Property	The grouping of numbers does not change the product.	$(2 \times 3) \times 4 = 2 \times (3 \times 4)$
Identity Property	Multiplying a number by one does not change its value.	$5 \times 1 = 5$
Zero Property	Multiplying a number by zero gives zero.	$7 \times 0 = 0$
Inverse Property	Multiplying a number by its reciprocal gives one.	$5 \times (1/5) = 1$
	Definition	Example

Understanding these properties allows for more efficient computation and a deeper comprehension of mathematical relationships.

Fractions, Decimals, and Percentages

Converting between fractions, decimals, and percentages is a critical skill in mathematics, especially in the context of the ATI TEAS exam. Each form presents a different way of representing parts of a whole, and knowing how to switch between them is essential.

Fractions

Fractions consist of a numerator and a denominator. They represent parts of a whole and can be classified as proper, improper, or mixed:

Type	Definition	Example
Proper Fraction	Numerator is less than the denominator.	3/4
Improper Fraction	Numerator is greater than or equal to the denominator.	5/4
Mixed Number	Combination of a whole number and a proper fraction.	1 1/2

Decimals

Decimals are another way of expressing fractions, using a decimal point to separate the whole number part from the fractional part:

Form	Example	Form
Terminating Decimal	0.75	Terminating Decimal
Repeating Decimal	0.333...	Repeating Decimal

Percentages

Percentages represent parts per hundred and are often used in practical contexts like discounts, interest rates, and statistics:

Form	Example	Form
Percentage	75%	Percentage

Converting Between Forms

Conversion between fractions, decimals, and percentages is often required. Here are the basic steps:

Conversion	Method	Conversion
Fraction to Decimal	Divide the numerator by the denominator.	Fraction to Decimal
Decimal to Percentage	Multiply by 100 and add the percent sign.	Decimal to Percentage
Percentage to Fraction	Write the percentage as a fraction with 100 as the denominator and simplify.	Percentage to Fraction

Ratios and Proportions

Ratios and proportions are tools for comparing quantities and understanding relationships between them. Ratios are expressed as fractions, while proportions are equations that state two ratios are equal.

Concept	Definition	Example
Ratio	A comparison of two quantities.	3:4 or 3/4
Proportion	An equation stating two ratios are equal.	3/4 = 6/8

Understanding how to work with ratios and proportions is vital for solving many types of mathematical problems, particularly those involving scale, rate, and comparison.

Algebraic Foundations

Algebra introduces variables and unknowns into mathematics, allowing for the expression of general relationships and the solving of equations. Key concepts include:

Variables represent unknown values and can be manipulated according to algebraic rules:

Concept	Definition	Example
Variable	A symbol representing an unknown value.	x, y
Algebraic Expression	A combination of variables, numbers, and operations.	2x + 3

Solving Equations

Equations are statements of equality that can be solved to find the value of the variables involved. The process involves isolating the variable on one side of the equation:

Step	Example	Step
Original Equation	$2x + 3 = 7$	Original Equation
Subtract 3 from both sides	$2x = 4$	Subtract 3 from both sides
Divide both sides by 2	$x = 2$	Divide both sides by 2

Geometry Basics

Geometry involves the study of shapes, sizes, and properties of space. Fundamental concepts include points, lines, angles, and shapes.

Points, Lines, and Angles

Concept	Definition	Example
Point	A location in space with no size.	.
Line	A collection of points extending infinitely in both directions.	---
Angle	Formed by two rays with a common endpoint.	$\angle ABC$

Shapes and Their Properties
Understanding the properties of different shapes is essential for solving geometric problems:

Shape	Properties	Shape
Triangle	Three sides, sum of angles is 180°.	Triangle
Square	Four equal sides, four right angles.	Square
Circle	All points equidistant from the center.	Circle

Measurement and Data

Measurement involves determining the size, length, or amount of something, while data involves collecting and analyzing information. Both are critical for practical applications of mathematics.

Type	Units
Length	Inches, feet, meters
Weight	Pounds, kilograms
Volume	Liters, gallons

Data can be represented in various forms to make it easier to understand and analyze:

Form	Example
Table	Organizes data in rows and columns.
Graph	Visual representation of data.

Building a strong foundation in these basic mathematical concepts is crucial for success in the ATI TEAS exam and beyond. Each topic forms a building block that supports more advanced concepts and problem-solving skills. Mastery of these fundamentals ensures a solid mathematical foundation, empowering you to tackle more complex topics with confidence and competence.

BASIC MATH SKILLS

Mathematics is a language of logic and precision, and the foundation of this language lies in basic arithmetic skills. Mastery of arithmetic not only facilitates everyday calculations but also underpins more advanced mathematical concepts. In this chapter, we will cover arithmetic essentials, mastering whole numbers and operations, delving into integers and their properties, unraveling prime numbers and factors, and finding the greatest common divisor (GCD) and least common multiple (LCM).

Arithmetic Essentials

Arithmetic is the branch of mathematics dealing with numbers and the basic operations: addition, subtraction, multiplication, and division. These operations form the building blocks for more complex problem-solving.

Addition and Subtraction

Addition involves combining quantities, while subtraction involves finding the difference between quantities. Here are some examples:

Addition Example:

```
  467
+ 385
------
  852
```

In this example, we add each column starting from the right. The units column gives us 7 + 5 = 12, we write down 2 and carry over 1. The tens column is 6 + 8 + 1 = 15, write down 5 and carry over 1. The hundreds column is 4 + 3 + 1 = 8.

Subtraction Example:

```
  742
- 458
------
  284
```

Here, we subtract each column starting from the right. If necessary, we borrow from the next column to the left.

Multiplication and Division

Multiplication is repeated addition, while division is finding how many times one number is contained within another.

Multiplication Example

```
  436
×   7
------
 3052
```

We multiply each digit of 436 by 7, starting from the right.

Division Example

$$387 \div 9 = 43$$

9 goes into 38 four times (since 9 × 4 = 36), subtract 36 from 38 to get 2, bring down the 7 to get 27, and 9 goes into 27 three times exactly.

Mastering Whole Numbers and Operations

Whole numbers include all positive numbers, including zero, without any fractional or decimal parts. Understanding how to operate with whole numbers is crucial.

Properties of Operations

Operations with whole numbers adhere to specific properties that simplify calculations:

- Commutative Property
  The order of addition or multiplication does not change the result (e.g., 4 + 5 = 5 + 4).

- Associative Property
  The grouping of numbers does not change the sum or product (e.g., (2 + 3) + 4 = 2 + (3 + 4)).

- Distributive Property
  Multiplying a number by a group of numbers added together is the same as doing each multiplication separately (e.g., 3 × (4 + 2) = (3 × 4) + (3 × 2)).

- Identity Property
  Adding 0 or multiplying by 1 does not change the value (e.g., 7 + 0 = 7, 5 × 1 = 5).

Working with Whole Numbers

To master whole numbers, practice these properties and ensure accuracy in calculations.

Example Problem:

Calculate: (5 + 3) × 4

Solution:
- Step 1: Add the numbers in parentheses:
  5 + 3 = 8
- Step 2: Multiply the result by 4:
  8 × 4 = 32

Delving into Integers and Their Properties

Integers expand the concept of whole numbers to include negative numbers, providing a complete picture of the number line.

Understanding Integers
Integers include all positive and negative whole numbers, along with zero. They are essential for expressing values below zero, such as temperatures and debts.

Properties of Integers
Integers follow similar properties as whole numbers, with additional considerations for negative values:

- Commutative Property
  Applies to both addition and multiplication.

- Associative Property
  Applies to both addition and multiplication.

- Distributive Property
  Applies to both positive and negative numbers.

- Additive Inverse
  The sum of an integer and its opposite is zero (e.g., 6 + (-6) = 0).

Example Problem:

- Calculate:
  -5 + 3 - (-2)
- Step 1: Add the first two numbers
  -5 + 3 = -2
- Step 2: Subtract the negative value (which is the same as adding its positive)
  -2 + 2 = 0

Unraveling Prime Numbers and Factors

Prime numbers and factors are fundamental concepts in number theory, crucial for various mathematical applications.

Prime Numbers
Prime numbers are numbers greater than 1 that have no positive divisors other than 1 and themselves. They are the building blocks of all numbers.

Examples of Prime Numbers:
2, 3, 5, 7, 11, 13, 17, 19, …

Factors

Factors are numbers that divide another number exactly without leaving a remainder. Every number has at least two factors: 1 and itself.
Example:
Factors of 12: 1, 2, 3, 4, 6, 12

Finding Factors

To find the factors of a number, start by dividing it by the smallest prime numbers and continue with the results.

Example Problem:

Find the factors of 28.
Solution:
- Step 1: Divide by 1: 28 ÷ 1 = 28
- Step 2: Divide by 2: 28 ÷ 2 = 14
- Step 3: Divide by 4: 28 ÷ 4 = 7
- Factors: 1, 2, 4, 7, 14, 28

Finding the Greatest Common Divisor and Least Common Multiple

The greatest common divisor (GCD) and least common multiple (LCM) are critical for simplifying fractions and solving problems involving multiple numbers.

Greatest Common Divisor (GCD)

The GCD of two numbers is the largest number that divides both of them without leaving a remainder. It is found using the Euclidean algorithm or by listing factors.

Example Problem:
Find the GCD of 48 and 64.
Solution:
- Step 1: List the factors of 48:
    1, 2, 3, 4, 6, 8, 12, 16, 24, 48
- Step 2: List the factors of 64:
    1, 2, 4, 8, 16, 32, 64
- Step 3: Identify the common factors:
    1, 2, 4, 8, 16
- GCD: 16

Least Common Multiple (LCM)

The LCM of two numbers is the smallest number that is a multiple of both. It can be found using prime factorization or listing multiples.

Example Problem:
Find the LCM of 12 and 15.
Solution:
- Step 1: List the multiples of 1212, 24, 36, 48, 60, 72, 84, 96, …
- Step 2: List the multiples of 15: 15, 30, 45, 60, 75, 90, 105, …
- Step 3: Identify the common multiples: 60, 120, …
- LCM: 60

Mastering these basic math skills provides a solid foundation for tackling more complex mathematical concepts and problems. Each section builds on the previous one, creating a cohesive understanding of arithmetic and its applications. Through practice and familiarity with these essentials, you will develop the confidence and competence needed for the ATI TEAS exam and beyond.

Tackling Advanced Mathematical Challenges is a journey that begins with a solid understanding of algebra, a branch of mathematics that uses symbols and letters to represent numbers and quantities in formulas and equations. This section will explore various aspects of algebra, from navigating algebraic expressions to understanding variables and constants, simplifying complex equations, decoding inequalities, and exploring exponents and radicals. Each concept will be thoroughly explained with numerous examples, word problems, and detailed solutions to ensure a deep understanding.

Deciphering Fractions and Decimals

Fractions and decimals are two ways of representing parts of a whole. Understanding their properties and how to work with them is crucial for solving a wide range of mathematical problems.

Understanding Fractions

A fraction consists of two parts: the numerator and the denominator. The numerator indicates how many parts are being considered, while the denominator indicates the total number of equal parts.

Examples:

- Proper Fractions: The numerator is less than the denominator (e.g., 3/4, 5/8).
- Improper Fractions: The numerator is greater than or equal to the denominator (e.g., 7/4, 9/8).
- Mixed Numbers: A whole number combined with a proper fraction (e.g., 2 1/2, 3 3/4).

Fractions can also be simplified by dividing both the numerator and the denominator by their greatest common divisor (GCD).

Example:
Simplify 18/24.

Solution: The GCD of 18 and 24 is 6.
18 ÷ 6 = 3
24 ÷ 6 = 4

So, 18/24 simplifies to 3/4.

Understanding Decimals

Decimals are another way to represent fractions, using a decimal point to separate the whole number part from the fractional part. Decimals are particularly useful in contexts where precise measurements are required.

Examples:

- Terminating Decimals: These have a finite number of digits after the decimal point (e.g., 0.75, 3.142).
- Repeating Decimals: These have one or more repeating digits after the decimal point (e.g., 0.333..., 1.666...).

Converting Fractions to Decimals

To convert a fraction to a decimal, divide the numerator by the denominator.

Example:
Convert 3/4 to a decimal.

Solution:
3 ÷ 4 = 0.75
So, 3/4 = 0.75.

Converting Decimals to Fractions

To convert a decimal to a fraction, place the decimal over 1 and multiply both the numerator and the denominator by 10 for each digit after the decimal point, then simplify if possible.

Example:
Convert 0.75 to a fraction.

Solution:
0.75 = 75/100
The GCD of 75 and 100 is 25.
75 ÷ 25 = 3
100 ÷ 25 = 4
So, 0.75 = 3/4.

Operations with Fractions and Decimals Simplified
Performing operations with fractions and decimals can be straightforward once you understand the rules and methods involved.

Adding and Subtracting Fractions

To add or subtract fractions, they must have a common denominator. Find the least common multiple (LCM) of the denominators, convert the fractions, and then add or subtract the numerators.

Example:
Add 1/4 and 2/3.

Solution:

The LCM of 4 and 3 is 12.
1/4 = 3/12
2/3 = 8/12
So, 1/4 + 2/3 = 3/12 + 8/12 = 11/12.

Multiplying and Dividing Fractions

To multiply fractions, multiply the numerators and denominators. To divide fractions, multiply by the reciprocal of the divisor.

Example:
Multiply 3/5 by 2/7.

Solution:
3/5 × 2/7 = 3 × 2 / 5 × 7 = 6/35.

Example:
Divide 3/5 by 2/7.

Solution:
3/5 ÷ 2/7 = 3/5 × 7/2 = 3 × 7 / 5 × 2 = 21/10 = 2 1/10.

Adding and Subtracting Decimals

Align the decimal points and add or subtract the numbers as if they were whole numbers.

Example:
Add 1.75 and 2.3.

Solution:
  1.75
+ 2.30

  4.05

Multiplying and Dividing Decimals

For multiplication, multiply as if there were no decimal points, then place the decimal point in the product so that the total number of decimal places is the sum of the decimal places in the factors.

Example:
Multiply 1.5 by 2.3.

Solution:
 1.5
× 2.3
------
 345 (1.5 × 2.3 = 3.45)

For division, move the decimal point in the divisor to the right end and move the decimal point in the dividend the same number of places. Then divide as with whole numbers.

Example:
Divide 4.5 by 1.5.
Solution:

4.5 ÷ 1.5 = 45 ÷ 15 = 3.

Harnessing the Power of Percentages

Percentages are a way of expressing parts per hundred and are useful for comparing quantities and understanding proportions.

Understanding Percentages

A percentage represents a fraction with a denominator of 100. It is often used in contexts such as discounts, interest rates, and data analysis.

Examples:

50% is equivalent to 50/100 or 1/2.
25% is equivalent to 25/100 or 1/4.

Calculating Percentages

To find a percentage of a number, multiply the number by the percentage and divide by 100.

Example:

Find 20% of 50.
Solution:
20% of 50 = 20/100 × 50 = 10.

Converting Between Percentages and Decimals

To convert a percentage to a decimal, divide by 100. To convert a decimal to a percentage, multiply by 100.

Example:
Convert 75% to a decimal.
Solution:
75% = 75/100 = 0.75.

Example:
Convert 0.85 to a percentage.
Solution:
0.85 × 100 = 85%.

Finding Percentage Increase or Decrease

To calculate the percentage increase or decrease, subtract the original value from the new value, divide by the original value, and multiply by 100.

Example:
Calculate the percentage increase from 40 to 50.
Solution:
Increase = 50 - 40 = 10
Percentage increase = (10 / 40) × 100 = 25%

Converting Between Fractions, Decimals, and Percentages Made Easy

Converting between fractions, decimals, and percentages is a fundamental skill that enables you to approach problems from different angles and contexts.

Fraction to Decimal Conversion

Divide the numerator by the denominator.

Example:
Convert 3/4 to a decimal.
Solution:
$3 \div 4 = 0.75$

Decimal to Fraction Conversion

Write the decimal as a fraction with a denominator of 10, 100, 1000, etc., depending on the number of decimal places, and simplify.

Example:
Convert 0.75 to a fraction.
Solution:
$0.75 = 75/100 = \frac{3}{4}$

Fraction to Percentage Conversion

Multiply the fraction by 100 and add the percent sign.

Example:
Convert 3/4 to a percentage.
Solution:
$3/4 \times 100 = 75\%$

Percentage to Fraction Conversion

Write the percentage as a fraction with a denominator of 100 and simplify.

Example:
Convert 75% to a fraction.
Solution:
$75\% = 75/100 = \frac{3}{4}$

Decimal to Percentage Conversion

Multiply the decimal by 100 and add the percent sign.

Example:
Convert 0.85 to a percentage.

Solution:
$0.85 \times 100 = 85\%$

Percentage to Decimal Conversion

Divide the percentage by 100.
Example:
Convert 60% to a decimal.
Solution:
$60\% = 60/100 = 0.60$

Practical Applications and Problem Solving

Understanding how to work with fractions, decimals, and percentages is crucial for solving real-world problems. Whether calculating discounts during shopping, understanding interest rates for loans, or analyzing data, these skills are indispensable.

Example Problem 1: Shopping Discount
A jacket is priced at $80, and there is a 25% discount. What is the sale price?

Solution:
Discount = 25% of $80 = 0.25×80 = $20
Sale price = $80 - $20 = $60

Example Problem 2: Interest Rate Calculation
If you invest $1000 at an annual interest rate of 5%, how much will you have after one year?

Interest = 5% of $1000 = 0.05×1000 = $50
Total amount after one year = $1000 + $50 = $1050

Example Problem 3: Data Analysis
A survey shows that 40% of participants prefer product A, 35% prefer product B, and the rest prefer product C. If 200 people participated in the survey, how many people prefer each product?

Solution:

Number of people preferring product A = 40% of 200 = 0.40 × 200 = 80

Number of people preferring product B = 35% of 200 = 0.35 × 200 = 70

Number of people preferring product C = 200 - (80 + 70) = 50

Example Problem 4: Baking Proportions

A recipe calls for 2/3 cup of sugar. If you want to make half of the recipe, how much sugar do you need?

Solution:

Sugar needed = 1/2 × 2/3 = 2/6 = 1/3 cup

Example Problem 5: Travel Distance

You traveled 250 miles, which is 5/8 of your total planned trip. How many miles is your total trip?

Solution:

Let the total trip distance be x.

5/8 of x = 250

x = 250 ÷ (5/8) = 250 × (8/5) = 400 miles

Tackling Advanced Mathematical Challenges requires a solid foundation in algebra, a branch of mathematics that uses symbols and letters to represent numbers and quantities in formulas and equations. Navigating Algebraic Expressions is the first step in this journey. Algebraic expressions are combinations of variables, constants, and operations that together create a mathematical phrase.

Tackling Advanced Mathematical Challenges is a journey that begins with a solid understanding of algebra, a branch of mathematics that uses symbols and letters to represent numbers and quantities in formulas and equations. This section will explore various aspects of algebra, from navigating algebraic expressions to understanding variables and constants, simplifying complex equations, decoding inequalities, and exploring exponents and radicals. Each concept will be thoroughly explained with numerous examples, word problems, and detailed solutions to ensure a deep understanding.

Navigating Algebraic Expressions

Algebraic expressions are combinations of variables, constants, and operations that together create a mathematical phrase. They form the foundation of algebra and are essential for understanding more complex mathematical concepts.

To begin with, consider the expression 4(2x + 3) - 5(3x - 2). To simplify this expression, we need to distribute the constants and then combine like terms. Here's how we do it:

Distribute the constants:
4 × 2x + 4 × 3 - 5 × 3x + 5 × 2
= 8x + 12 - 15x + 10

Combine like terms:
8x - 15x + 12 + 10
= -7x + 22

Simplifying algebraic expressions often involves recognizing and applying the distributive property, combining like terms, and

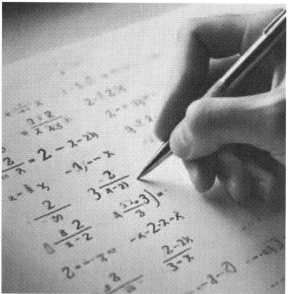

understanding the role of coefficients and variables.

Another example is simplifying the expression 3(a + b) - 2(a - b). First, distribute the constants:

3a + 3b - 2a + 2b

Next, combine like terms:

(3a - 2a) + (3b + 2b)
= a + 5b

Through these examples, we see that navigating algebraic expressions requires careful application of basic algebraic rules and properties.

Understanding Variables and Constants

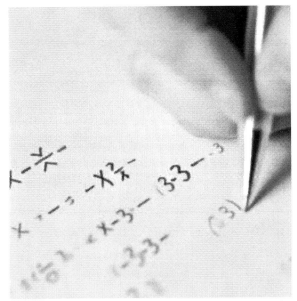

Variables are symbols, often letters, that represent numbers whose values are not yet known. Constants, on the other hand, are fixed values that do not change. Understanding the difference between these two is crucial for solving algebraic equations.

Consider the equation 3x - 7 = 2x + 5. Here, 'x' is the variable, and the numbers 3, -7, 2, and 5 are constants. To solve for x, we need to isolate the variable on one side of the equation. Here's the step-by-step process:

Subtract 2x from both sides to get the variables on one side:
3x - 2x - 7 = 5

Combine like terms:
x - 7 = 5

Add 7 to both sides to isolate x:
x = 12

This process involves understanding how to manipulate variables and constants to find the value of the unknown variable.

Another example involves a real-life scenario. Suppose a car rental company charges a base fee of $50 per day plus $0.20 per mile driven. To write an expression for the total cost C of renting a car for one day and driving x miles, we can use the following formula:

C = 50 + 0.20x

Here, C is the total cost (variable), 50 is the base fee (constant), and 0.20x represents the mileage fee (variable depending on x).

These examples illustrate how understanding variables and constants is essential for modeling real-world situations and solving equations.

Simplifying Complex Equations with Ease

Equations are mathematical statements that assert the equality of two expressions. They often include variables, and the goal is to find the values of these variables that make the equation true. Simplifying complex equations involves combining like terms, using the distributive property, and applying inverse operations.

Consider the equation 2(3x + 4) - 5x = 7. To simplify, we first distribute the 2:

6x + 8 - 5x = 7

Next, combine like terms:

x + 8 = 7

34

Finally, isolate the variable by subtracting 8 from both sides:

x = -1

This process requires attention to detail and a systematic approach to solving equations.

Let's look at another example. Solve the equation 4x - 5(2 - x) = 3x + 7. Start by distributing the -5:

4x - 10 + 5x = 3x + 7

Combine like terms:

9x - 10 = 3x + 7

Subtract 3x from both sides to get the variables on one side:

6x - 10 = 7

Add 10 to both sides:

6x = 17

Divide both sides by 6:

x = 17/6 or approximately 2.83

Through these examples, we see that simplifying complex equations involves using algebraic properties and operations to isolate the variable and solve for its value.

Word problems often provide practical applications of these skills. For example, the sum of three consecutive integers is 51. Find the integers.

Let the first integer be x. Then the next two integers are x + 1 and x + 2. The sum of these integers is:

x + (x + 1) + (x + 2) = 51

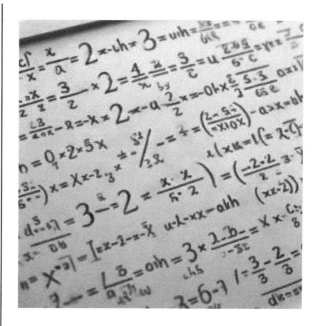

Combine like terms:

3x + 3 = 51

Subtract 3 from both sides:

3x = 48

Divide by 3:

x = 16

So, the integers are 16, 17, and 18.

This word problem demonstrates how to apply algebraic techniques to find unknown values in real-life scenarios.

Decoding Inequalities

Inequalities are statements that compare two expressions. Unlike equations, inequalities show that one expression is greater than, less than, greater than or equal to, or less than or equal to another. Solving inequalities often involves similar steps to solving equations but requires careful consideration of the inequality's direction, especially when multiplying or dividing by a negative number.

Consider the inequality $3x - 4 \leq 2x + 5$. To solve, we first subtract $2x$ from both sides:

$x - 4 \leq 5$

Next, add 4 to both sides:

$x \leq 9$

This solution means that x can be any number less than or equal to 9.

Another example is solving the inequality $-2(x - 3) > 4$. Start by distributing the -2:

$-2x + 6 > 4$

Subtract 6 from both sides:

$-2x > -2$

Divide both sides by -2 (and remember to reverse the inequality sign):

$x < 1$

This solution means that x can be any number less than 1.

Word problems also frequently involve inequalities. For instance, a student needs at least 75 points to pass a test. If the test has 100 questions and each question is worth 1 point, write an inequality to represent the minimum number of questions the student must answer correctly to pass.

Let x represent the number of questions answered correctly. The inequality is:

$x \geq 75$

This inequality shows that the student must answer at least 75 questions correctly to pass the test.

Exploring Exponents and Radicals

Exponents represent repeated multiplication of a base number. For example, 2^3 means 2 multiplied by itself three times: $2 \times 2 \times 2 = 8$. Radicals, such as square roots, represent the inverse operation. The square root of 9, written as $\sqrt{9}$, is 3 because $3 \times 3 = 9$.

Consider the equation $x^2 - 5x + 6 = 0$. To solve, factor the quadratic expression:

$(x - 2)(x - 3) = 0$

This gives two solutions:

$x = 2$ and $x = 3$

These values are the roots of the equation.

Another example involves simplifying the expression $(2^3)^2$. Apply the power of a power rule (multiply the exponents):

$(2^3)^2 = 2^{(3 \times 2)} = 2^6 = 64$

Let's look at a practical application. A scientist observes that a certain bacteria population doubles every hour. If the initial population is 500, write an expression for the population after t hours and find the population after 5 hours.

The population P after t hours is given by:

$P = 500 \times 2^t$

For $t = 5$:

$P = 500 \times 2^5 = 500 \times 32 = 16000$

These examples illustrate the importance of understanding and applying the properties of exponents and radicals to solve problems effectively.

As we continue to explore these topics, it's important to practice regularly and apply these concepts to a variety of problems. By doing so, Let's delve deeper into each of these areas with more examples, word problem
and detailed solutions to further solidify your understanding

.

you will develop a deeper understanding and greater confidence in your mathematical abilities. This will not only prepare you for exams but also enhance your problem-solving skills in everyday life.

Navigating Algebraic Expressions

Example: Simplify the expression 5(2x - 3) + 4(3x + 1).
Solution: Distribute the constants:
$5 \times 2x - 5 \times 3 + 4 \times 3x + 4 \times 1$
$= 10x - 15 + 12x + 4$

Combine like terms:
$10x + 12x - 15 + 4$
$= 22x - 11$

Simplifying algebraic expressions often involves recognizing and applying the distributive property, combining like terms, and understanding the role of coefficients and variables.

Another example is simplifying the expression 4(a - b) - 3(b - a). First, distribute the constants:

$4a - 4b - 3b + 3a$

Next, combine like terms:

$(4a + 3a) - (4b + 3b)$
$= 7a - 7b$

Through these examples, we see that navigating algebraic expressions requires careful application of basic algebraic rules and properties.

Understanding Variables and Constants

Example: If 4x - 8 = 2x + 10, find the value of x.
Solution: Subtract 2x from both sides to get the variables on one side:
$4x - 2x - 8 = 10$

Combine like terms:
$2x - 8 = 10$

Add 8 to both sides to isolate x:

$2x = 18$

Divide by 2:
$x = 9$

This process involves understanding how to manipulate variables and constants to find the value of the unknown variable.

Another example involves a real-life scenario. Suppose a taxi company charges a base fee of $3 plus $2 per mile driven. To write an expression for the total cost C of a taxi ride for m miles, we can use the following formula:

$C = 3 + 2m$

Here, C is the total cost (variable), 3 is the base fee (constant), and 2m represents the mileage fee (variable depending on m).

These examples illustrate how understanding variables and constants is essential for modeling real-world situations and solving equations.

Simplifying Complex Equations with Ease

Example: Solve the equation 5x - 3(2x + 4) = 7. To simplify, we first distribute the -3:

$5x - 6x - 12 = 7$

Next, combine like terms:

$-x - 12 = 7$

Add 12 to both sides to isolate the variable:

$-x = 19$

Multiply both sides by -1:

$x = -19$

This process requires attention to detail and a systematic approach to solving equations.

Let's look at another example. Solve the equation 3(2x - 1) = 4(x + 5). Start by distributing the constants:

6x - 3 = 4x + 20

Subtract 4x from both sides to get the variables on one side:

2x - 3 = 20

Add 3 to both sides:

2x = 23

Divide by 2:

x = 23/2 or 11.5

Through these examples, we see that simplifying complex equations involves using algebraic properties and operations to isolate the variable and solve for its value.

Word problems often provide practical applications of these skills. For example, the sum of four consecutive even integers is 60. Find the integers.

Let the first even integer be x. Then the next three even integers are x + 2, x + 4, and x + 6. The sum of these integers is:

x + (x + 2) + (x + 4) + (x + 6) = 60

Combine like terms:

4x + 12 = 60

Subtract 12 from both sides:

4x = 48

Divide by 4:

x = 12

So, the integers are 12, 14, 16, and 18.

This word problem demonstrates how to apply algebraic techniques to find unknown values in real-life scenarios.

Decoding Inequalities

Example: Solve the inequality 4x - 5 > 2x + 3.
Solution: Subtract 2x from both sides to get the variables on one side:
4x - 2x - 5 > 3

Combine like terms:
2x - 5 > 3

Add 5 to both sides:
2x > 8

Divide by 2:
x > 4

This solution means that x can be any number greater than 4.

Another example is solving the inequality -3(x - 2) ≤ 9. Start by distributing the -3:

-3x + 6 ≤ 9

Subtract 6 from both sides:

-3x ≤ 3

Divide both sides by -3 (and remember to reverse the inequality sign):

x ≥ -1

properties and operations to isolate the variable and solve for its value.

Word problems often provide practical applications of these skills. For example, the sum of five consecutive odd integers is 65. Find the integers.

Let the first odd integer be x. Then the next four odd integers are x + 2, x + 4, x + 6, and x + 8. The sum of these integers is:

x + (x + 2) + (x + 4) + (x + 6) + (x + 8) = 65

Combine like terms:

5x + 20 = 65

Subtract 20 from both sides:

5x = 45

Divide by 5:

x = 9

So, the integers are 9, 11, 13, 15, and 17.

This word problem demonstrates how to apply algebraic techniques to find unknown values in real-life scenarios.

Decoding Inequalities

Example: Solve the inequality 5x - 7 ≥ 2x + 4.
Solution: Subtract 2x from both sides to get the variables on one side:
5x - 2x - 7 ≥ 4

Combine like terms:
3x - 7 ≥ 4

Add 7 to both sides:
3x ≥ 11

Divide by 3:
x ≥ 11/3 or approximately 3.67

This solution means that x can be any number greater than or equal to 3.67.

Another example is solving the inequality -4(x - 1) < 8. Start by distributing the -4:

-4x + 4 < 8

Subtract 4 from both sides:

-4x < 4

Divide both sides by -4 (and remember to reverse the inequality sign):

x > -1

This solution means that x can be any number greater than -1.

Word problems also frequently involve inequalities. For instance, a factory needs to produce at least 1000 units of a product each week to meet orders. If the factory operates 5 days a week and produces x units per day, write an inequality to represent the minimum number of units produced per day to meet the weekly target.

The inequality is:

5x ≥ 1000

Divide both sides by 5:

x ≥ 200

This inequality shows that the factory must produce at least 200 units per day to meet the weekly target.

Exploring Exponents and Radicals

Exponents represent repeated multiplication of a base number. For example, 2^3 means 2 multiplied by itself three times: $2 \times 2 \times 2 = 8$. Radicals, such as square roots, represent the inverse operation. The square root of 9, written as $\sqrt{9}$, is 3 because $3 \times 3 = 9$.

Consider the equation $x^2 - 5x + 6 = 0$. To solve, factor the quadratic expression:

$(x - 2)(x - 3) = 0$

This gives two solutions:

$x = 2$ and $x = 3$

These values are the roots of the equation.

Another example involves simplifying the expression $(2^3)^2$. Apply the power of a power rule (multiply the exponents):

$(2^3)^2 = 2^{(3 \times 2)} = 2^6 = 64$

Let's look at a practical application. A scientist observes that a certain bacteria population doubles every hour. If the initial population is 500, write an expression for the population after t hours and find the population after 5 hours.

The population P after t hours is given by:

$P = 500 \times 2^t$

For $t = 5$:

$P = 500 \times 2^5 = 500 \times 32 = 16000$

These examples illustrate the importance of understanding and applying the properties of exponents and radicals to solve problems effectively.

As we continue to explore these topics, it's important to practice regularly and apply these concepts to a variety of problems. By doing so, you will develop a deeper understanding and greater confidence in your mathematical abilities. This will not only prepare you for exams but also enhance your problem-solving skills in everyday life.

Let's delve deeper into each of these areas with more examples, word problems, and detailed solutions to further solidify your understanding.

Navigating Algebraic Expressions

Example: Simplify the expression $5(2x - 3) + 4(3x + 1)$.
Solution: Distribute the constants:
$5 \times 2x - 5 \times 3 + 4 \times 3x + 4 \times 1$
$= 10x - 15 + 12x + 4$

Combine like terms:
$10x + 12x - 15 + 4$
$= 22x - 11$

Simplifying algebraic expressions often involves recognizing and applying the distributive property, combining like terms, and understanding the role of coefficients and variables.

Another example is simplifying the expression $4(a - b) - 3(b - a)$. First, distribute the constants:

$4a - 4b - 3b + 3a$

Next, combine like terms:

$(4a + 3a) - (4b + 3b)$
$= 7a - 7b$

Through these examples, we see that navigating algebraic expressions requires careful application of basic algebraic rules and properties.

Understanding Variables and Constants

Example: If $4x - 8 = 2x + 10$, find the value of x.
Solution: Subtract 2x from both sides to get the variables on one side:
$4x - 2x - 8 = 10$

Combine like terms:
$2x - 8 = 10$

Add 8 to both sides to isolate x:
$2x = 18$

Divide by 2:
$x = 9$

This process involves understanding how to manipulate variables and constants to find the value of the unknown variable.

Another example involves a real-life scenario. Suppose a taxi company charges a base fee of $3 plus $2 per mile driven. To write an expression for the total cost C of a taxi ride for m miles, we can use the following formula:

$C = 3 + 2m$

Here, C is the total cost (variable), 3 is the base fee (constant), and 2m represents the mileage fee (variable depending on m).

These examples illustrate how understanding variables and constants is essential for modeling real-world situations and solving equations.

Simplifying Complex Equations with Ease

Example: Solve the equation $5x - 3(2x + 4) = 7$. To simplify, we first distribute the -3:

$5x - 6x - 12 = 7$

Next, combine like terms:

$-x - 12 = 7$

Add 12 to both sides to isolate the variable:

$-x = 19$

Multiply both sides by -1:

$x = -19$

This process requires attention to detail and a systematic approach to solving equations.

Let's look at another example. Solve the equation $3(2x - 1) = 4(x + 5)$. Start by distributing the constants:

$6x - 3 = 4x + 20$

Subtract 4x from both sides to get the variables on one side:

$2x - 3 = 20$

Add 3 to both sides:

$2x = 23$

Divide by 2:
$x = 23/2$ or 11.5

Through these examples, we see that simplifying complex equations involves using algebraic properties and operations to isolate the variable and solve for its value.

Word problems often provide practical applications of these skills. For example, the sum of four consecutive even integers is 60. Find the integers.

Let the first even integer be x. Then the next three even integers are $x + 2$, $x + 4$, and $x + 6$. The sum of these integers is:

x + (x + 2) + (x + 4) + (x + 6) = 60

Combine like terms:

4x + 12 = 60
Subtract 12 from both sides:

4x = 48

Divide by 4:

x = 12

So, the integers are 12, 14, 16, and 18.

This word problem demonstrates how to apply algebraic techniques to find unknown values in real-life scenarios.

Decoding Inequalities

Example: Solve the inequality $4x - 5 > 2x + 3$.
Solution: Subtract 2x from both sides to get the variables on one side:
$4x - 2x - 5 > 3$

Combine like terms:
$2x - 5 > 3$

Add 5 to both sides:
$2x > 8$

Divide by 2:
$x > 4$

This solution means that x can be any number greater than 4.

Another example is solving the inequality $-3(x - 2) \leq 9$. Start by distributing the -3:

$-3x + 6 \leq 9$

Subtract 6 from both sides:

$-3x \leq 3$
Divide both sides by -3 (and remember to reverse the inequality sign):

$x \geq -1$

This solution means that x can be any number greater than or equal to -1.

Word problems also frequently involve inequalities. For instance, a company needs to produce at least 500 units of a product to meet demand. If the company can produce 50 units per day, write an inequality to represent the minimum number of days d the company must operate to meet the demand.

The inequality is:

$50d \geq 500$

Divide both sides by 50:
$d \geq 10$

This inequality shows that the company must operate for at least 10 days to meet the demand.

Exploring Exponents and Radicals

Example: Simplify the expression $(3^2)^3$.
Solution: Apply the power of a power rule (multiply the exponents):

$(3^2)^3 = 3^{(2 \times 3)} = 3^6 = 729$

Another example involves solving the equation $4x^2 - 16 = 0$. Start by isolating the term with the exponent:

$4x^2 = 16$

Divide by 4:

$x^2 = 4$

Take the square root of both sides:

x = ±2

This solution means that x can be either 2 or -2.

Let's look at a practical application. A population of bacteria triples every hour. If the initial population is 200, write an expression for the population after t hours and find the population after 4 hours.

The population P after t hours is given by:

$P = 200 \times 3^t$

For t = 4:

$P = 200 \times 3^4 = 200 \times 81 = 16200$

These examples illustrate the importance of understanding and applying the properties of exponents and radicals to solve problems effectively.

As we continue to explore these topics, it's important to practice regularly and apply these concepts to a variety of problems. By doing so, you will develop a deeper understanding and greater confidence in your mathematical abilities. This will not only prepare you for exams but also enhance your problem-solving skills in everyday life.

greater confidence in your mathematical abilities. This will not only prepare you for exams but also enhance your problem-solving skills in everyday life.

Mathematics is not just a subject confined to textbooks and classrooms; it is a vital tool used in various aspects of everyday life. From budgeting and cooking to shopping and planning trips, mathematical principles underpin many daily activities. This section will explore the practical applications of mathematics, focusing on real-world math applications, mastering measurement and estimation techniques, visualizing data and statistics, interpreting graphs and charts, and grasping probability and basic statistics.

Real-world Math Applications

Math is integral to numerous real-world scenarios. For instance, when shopping, you might need to calculate discounts, compare prices, or budget your expenses. Consider the following example:

Example: Shopping Discount

A jacket originally costs $120, but it is on sale for 25% off. What is the sale price of the jacket?

Solution:
First, calculate the discount amount:
Discount = 25% of $120
Discount = 0.25 × 120
Discount = $30

Next, subtract the discount from the original price:
Sale Price = Original Price - Discount
Sale Price = $120 - $30
Sale Price = $90

In this example, the sale price of the jacket is $90. This type of problem demonstrates the importance of understanding percentages and basic arithmetic operations in everyday life.

Another common application of math is in cooking, where precise measurements are crucial for following recipes. Let's consider an example involving recipe adjustments:

Example: Recipe Adjustment

A cookie recipe calls for 2 cups of flour to make 24 cookies. How much flour is needed to make 36 cookies?

Solution:
First, determine the flour required for one cookie:
Flour per cookie = 2 cups / 24 cookies
Flour per cookie = 1/12 cups

Next, calculate the flour needed for 36 cookies:
Flour for 36 cookies = 1/12 cups × 36
Flour for 36 cookies = 3 cups

In this example, you need 3 cups of flour to make 36 cookies. This illustrates the application of ratios and proportions in cooking.

Mastering Measurement and Estimation Techniques

Measurement and estimation are essential skills in various fields, from construction and engineering to everyday tasks like home improvement and gardening. Accurate measurement ensures precision, while estimation helps make quick, reasonable judgments when exact values are not necessary.

Example: Room Painting

You want to paint the walls of a room that is 12 feet long, 10 feet wide, and 8 feet high. How much paint is needed if one gallon covers 350 square feet?

Solution:
First, calculate the total wall area:
Wall Area = 2(length × height) + 2(width × height)
Wall Area = 2(12 ft × 8 ft) + 2(10 ft × 8 ft)
Wall Area = 2(96 ft^2) + 2(80 ft^2)
Wall Area = 192 ft^2 + 160 ft^2
Wall Area = 352 ft^2

Next, determine the number of gallons needed:

Gallons Needed = Total Wall Area / Coverage per Gallon
Gallons Needed = 352 ft^2 / 350 ft^2/gallon
Gallons Needed ≈ 1.01 gallons

Since you can't purchase a fraction of a gallon, you would need to buy 2 gallons of paint to cover the room. This example demonstrates the practical application of area calculations and estimation.

Example: Garden Planning

You want to plant a rectangular garden that is 15 feet long and 10 feet wide. You plan to plant one tomato plant per square foot. How many tomato plants do you need?

Solution:
Calculate the area of the garden:
Garden Area = length × width
Garden Area = 15 ft × 10 ft

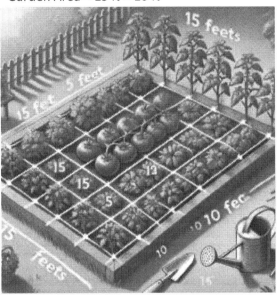

Garden Area = 150 ft^2

Since you plan to plant one tomato plant per square foot, you will need 150 tomato plants for your garden. This example shows how area calculations are used in gardening and planning.

Visualizing Data and Statistics

Data visualization is a powerful tool for understanding and interpreting data. Graphs, charts, and tables allow us to see patterns, trends, and relationships that might not be immediately apparent from raw data. Here are some common types of data visualization and their practical applications:

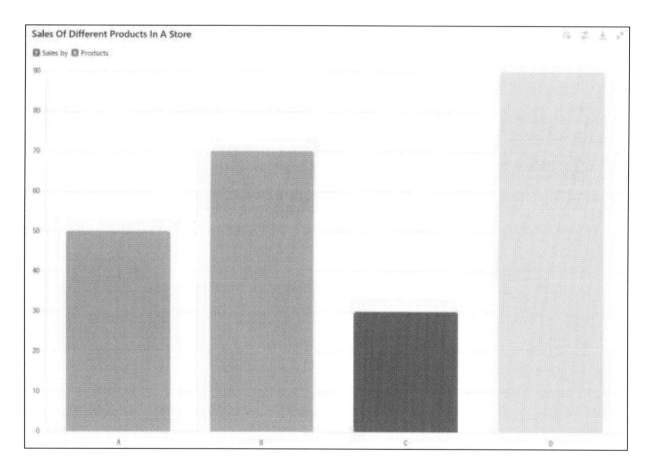

Example: Bar Graph

A bar graph is useful for comparing quantities across different categories. Suppose you are comparing the sales of different products in a store.

Products: A, B, C, D
Sales: 50, 70, 30, 90

Solution:
Draw a bar graph with the products on the x-axis and sales on the y-axis. Each bar represents the sales of a product.

Product A: 50
Product B: 70
Product C: 30

Product D: 90

The bar graph clearly shows that Product D has the highest sales, followed by Product B, Product A, and Product C. This type of visualization helps identify which products are performing well and which are not.

Example: Pie Chart

A pie chart is useful for showing the proportions of different categories within a whole. Suppose you are analyzing the budget allocation for a project.

Categories: Research, Development, Marketing, Operations
Budget Allocation: 20%, 30%, 25%, 25%

Solution:
Draw a pie chart with each category represented as a slice of the pie. The size of each slice corresponds to the budget allocation.

Research: 20%
Development: 30%
Marketing: 25%
Operations: 25%

The pie chart visually represents the budget allocation, making it easy to see that Development receives the largest share of the budget, followed by Marketing and Operations, with Research receiving the smallest share.

Example: Line Graph

A line graph is useful for showing trends over time. Suppose you are tracking the monthly sales of a product over a year.

Months: Jan, Feb, Mar, Apr, May, Jun, Jul, Aug, Sep, Oct, Nov, Dec
Sales: 100, 120, 130, 110, 150, 140, 160, 170, 180, 190, 200, 210

Solution:
Draw a line graph with months on the x-axis and sales on the y-axis. Plot each month's sales as a point and connect the points with a line.

The line graph shows the trend of increasing sales over the year, with a slight dip in April. This type of visualization helps identify trends and patterns in data over time.

Interpreting Graphs and Charts

Interpreting graphs and charts is an essential skill for understanding data and making informed decisions. Let's explore some examples:

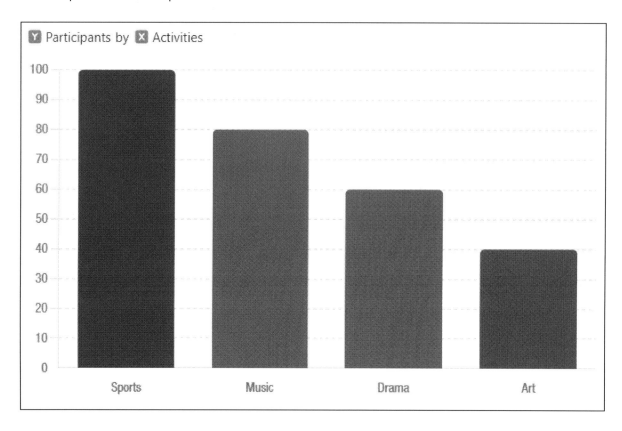

Example: Interpreting a Bar Graph

Suppose a bar graph shows the number of students participating in different extracurricular activities at a school.

Activities: Sports, Music, Drama, Art
Participants: 100, 80, 60, 40

Solution:
From the bar graph, you can see that Sports has the highest number of participants, followed by Music, Drama, and Art. This information can help the school allocate resources and support for each activity based on participation.

Example: Interpreting a Pie Chart

Suppose a pie chart shows the distribution of a company's expenses.

Categories: Salaries, Rent, Utilities, Supplies
Expenses: 40%, 25%, 20%, 15%

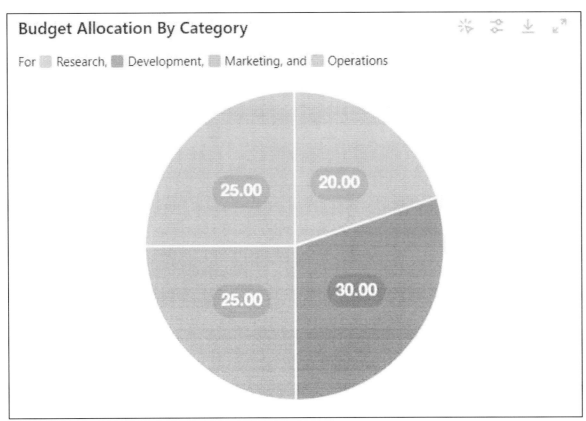

Budget Allocation By Category

For ▨ Research, ▮ Development, ▨ Marketing, and ▨ Operations

25.00   20.00

25.00   30.00

Solution:
The pie chart shows that Salaries account for the largest portion of the company's expenses, followed by Rent, Utilities, and Supplies. This information can help the company identify major expense categories and plan for cost management.

Example: Interpreting a Line Graph

Suppose a line graph shows the temperature changes over a week.

Days: Mon, Tue, Wed, Thu, Fri, Sat, Sun
Temperature (°F): 70, 72, 68, 65, 75, 78, 80

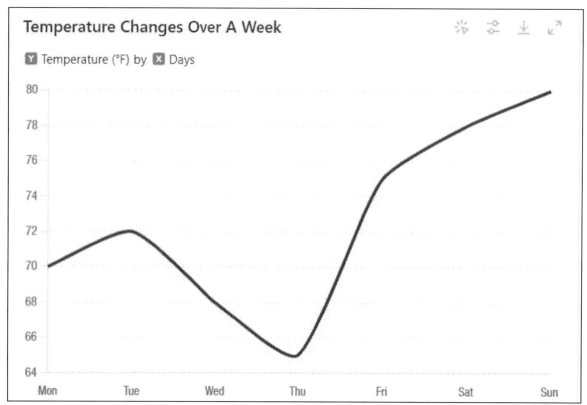

Temperature Changes Over A Week

Temperature (°F) by Days

Solution:

The line graph shows the temperature rising steadily from Thursday to Sunday, with a peak on Sunday. This information can help in planning outdoor activities based on temperature trends

Probability and statistics are essential for understanding and analyzing data, making predictions, and making informed decisions. Let's explore some basic concepts and their practical applications:

Probability

Probability is the measure of the likelihood of an event occurring. Suppose you have a fair six-sided die. What is the probability of rolling a 4?

Solution:

There are 6 possible outcomes when rolling a die, and only one of them is a 4. Therefore, the probability of rolling a 4 is:

P(rolling a 4) = 1/6 ≈ 0.167 or 16.7%

This example illustrates the basic concept of probability and how it is calculated.

Mean, Median, and Mode

The mean, median, and mode are measures of central tendency that summarize a set of data.

Suppose you have the following test scores: 85, 90, 78, 92, 88

Solution:
Mean (average) is calculated by adding all the scores and dividing by the number of scores:
Mean = (85 + 90 + 78 + 92 + 88) / 5
Mean = 433 / 5
Mean = 86.6

Median is the middle value when the scores are arranged in ascending order:
Scores in ascending order: 78, 85, 88, 90, 92
Median = 88

Mode is the most frequently occurring score. In this case, there is no mode because all scores occur only once.

These measures provide a summary of the data set, helping to understand the distribution of test scores.

Standard Deviation

Standard deviation measures the spread of data around the mean. Suppose you have the following weights (in kg) of 5 people: 60, 62, 65, 63, 61

Solution:
First, calculate the mean weight:
Mean = (60 + 62 + 65 + 63 + 61) / 5
Mean = 311 / 5
Mean = 62.2

Next, calculate the squared differences from the mean and the variance:

- Variance = $[(60 - 62.2)^2 + (62 - 62.2)^2 + (65 - 62.2)^2 + (63 - 62.2)^2 + (61 - 62.2)^2] / 5$
- Variance = $[(-2.2)^2 + (-0.2)^2 + (2.8)^2 + (0.8)^2 + (-1.2)^2] / 5$
- Variance = $[4.84 + 0.04 + 7.84 + 0.64 + 1.44] / 5$
- Variance = 14.8 / 5
- Variance = 2.96

Standard Deviation = √Variance
Standard Deviation = √2.96
Standard Deviation ≈ 1.72

The standard deviation of approximately 1.72 kg indicates the average amount by which individual weights differ from the mean weight.

Probability in Real-life Scenarios

Suppose you are planning an event and there is a 30% chance of rain. What is the probability that it will not rain?

Solution:
The probability of not raining is the complement of the probability of raining. Therefore:
P(not raining) = 1 - P(raining)
P(not raining) = 1 - 0.30
P(not raining) = 0.70 or 70%

This example shows how probability is used in making decisions based on uncertain outcomes.

Applying Basic Statistics to Business

A company wants to analyze the performance of its sales team. The sales data (in units sold) for the past five months are: 120, 150, 130, 140, 160

Solution:
First, calculate the mean sales:
Mean = (120 + 150 + 130 + 140 + 160) / 5
Mean = 700 / 5
Mean = 140

Next, calculate the median sales:
Sales in ascending order: 120, 130, 140, 150, 160
Median = 140

Finally, determine if there is a mode:
There is no mode because all sales figures occur only once.

The mean and median sales provide insight into the typical performance of the sales team, while the absence of a mode indicates no repeated sales figure.

Interpreting Statistical Results

Suppose you conducted a survey to determine the preferred mode of transportation among 100 people. The results are as follows:

Car: 40
Bike: 25
Public Transport: 20
Walking: 15

Solution:
To visualize this data, you can create a bar graph or pie chart. For the pie chart:
Car: 40%
Bike: 25%
Public Transport: 20%
Walking: 15%

Interpreting this data helps understand the most preferred mode of transportation (Car) and the least preferred (Walking). This information can be useful for urban planning and transportation services.

Probability in Games of Chance

Suppose you are playing a card game with a standard deck of 52 cards. What is the probability of drawing an Ace?

Solution:
There are 4 Aces in a deck of 52 cards. Therefore, the probability of drawing an Ace is:

P(drawing an Ace) = 4/52
P(drawing an Ace) = 1/13 ≈ 0.077 or 7.7%

This example illustrates the application of probability in games of chance, helping players understand their odds of winning.

In conclusion, mathematics is an indispensable tool that permeates various aspects of everyday life. From calculating discounts and adjusting recipes to planning events and analyzing data, mathematical principles are essential for making informed decisions and solving real-world problems. By mastering measurement and estimation techniques, visualizing data, interpreting graphs and charts, and understanding probability and basic statistics, you can develop a strong foundation in practical mathematics, enhancing your problem-solving skills and overall mathematical literacy. Regular practice and application of these concepts will not only prepare you for exams but also empower you to navigate and succeed in various real-life scenarios with confidence and competence.

HUMAN ANATOMY AND PHYSIOLOGY

Human anatomy and physiology form the cornerstone of our understanding of the human body, illuminating the intricate and dynamic structures and functions that sustain life. Anatomy delves into the physical architecture of the body, from the macroscopic bones and muscles to the microscopic cells and tissues, revealing a complex network of interconnected systems. Physiology, on the other hand, explores the mechanisms and processes that enable these structures to function cohesively, ensuring survival and homeostasis. Together, these fields offer a comprehensive view of how our bodies operate, adapt, and interact with the environment, providing invaluable insights into health, disease, and the remarkable resilience of the human organism.

The Cellular Level: Building Blocks of Life

Cells are the fundamental units of life, the smallest entities that can carry out all the processes necessary for life. Each cell functions as a tiny, self-contained factory, capable of generating energy, synthesizing proteins, and replicating itself. Within the human body, cells come in a multitude of shapes and sizes, each specialized for a unique function. For instance, red blood cells are shaped like discs to maximize surface area for oxygen transport, while nerve cells have long extensions to transmit electrical signals over distances.

The cell membrane, a phospholipid bilayer embedded with proteins, serves as the gatekeeper, regulating the movement of substances in and out of the cell. Within the membrane, the cytoplasm hosts various organelles, each performing specific tasks. The nucleus, often regarded as the control center, houses DNA, the blueprint of life. Ribosomes, either free-floating or attached to the endoplasmic reticulum, are the sites of protein synthesis. The mitochondria, known as the powerhouses of the cell, generate ATP through cellular respiration, a process involving the conversion of glucose and oxygen into energy.

Furthermore, the cellular level includes a myriad of processes such as mitosis and meiosis, which ensure cell division and genetic diversity, respectively. These processes are meticulously regulated by the cell cycle, involving phases like interphase, where the cell prepares for division, and mitosis, where the actual division occurs. Specialized cells form tissues, which in turn create organs, and eventually, organ systems. The intricate interplay between these components sustains life and supports the organism's growth, repair, and adaptation to environmental changes.

Tissues and Organs: Their Roles and Functions

Tissues are groups of similar cells working together to perform a specific function. There are four primary types of tissues in the human body: epithelial, connective, muscle, and nervous tissue. Epithelial tissue covers body surfaces and lines cavities, acting as a barrier and involved in absorption, secretion, and sensation. Connective tissue provides support and binds other tissues together; it includes bone, blood, and adipose tissue.

Muscle tissue is responsible for movement and is classified into three types: skeletal, cardiac, and smooth. Skeletal muscle is voluntary and striated, attached to bones to facilitate movement. Cardiac muscle, found only in the heart, is involuntary and striated, enabling the heart to pump blood. Smooth muscle, also involuntary, is found in walls of hollow organs like the intestines and blood vessels, where it regulates the flow of substances through these structures.

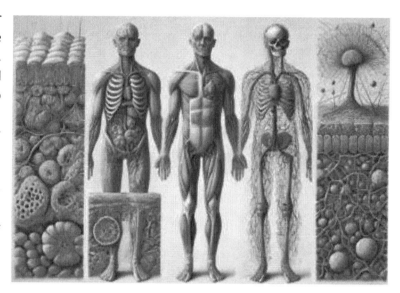

Nervous tissue consists of neurons and supporting glial cells, forming the nervous system which controls and coordinates body activities. Neurons transmit electrical impulses, while glial cells provide support and protection. These tissues combine to form organs, each performing specific functions essential to the body's operation. For instance, the stomach, an organ in the digestive system, consists of muscle tissue for churning food, epithelial tissue for lining, and connective tissue for structural support.

Organs interact within organ systems to maintain the body's overall function and homeostasis. The heart pumps blood through the vascular system, lungs facilitate gas exchange, and kidneys filter waste from the blood. Each organ system relies on the coordinated activity of its constituent tissues and organs to perform its role effectively, ensuring the body operates as a cohesive unit.

Systems of the Body: An Integrated Overview

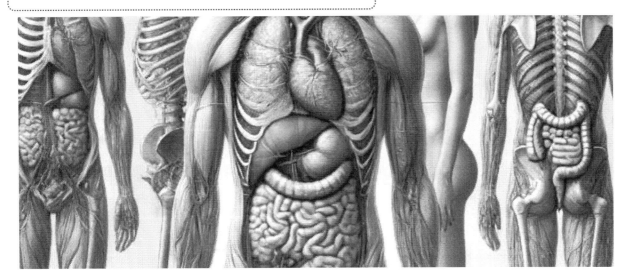

The human body comprises several interrelated systems, each with unique functions but all working in harmony to sustain life. These systems include the cardiovascular, respiratory, digestive, nervous, musculoskeletal, immune, endocrine, urinary, and reproductive systems. Each system relies on others to perform its role effectively. For instance, the respiratory system supplies oxygen to the blood, which the cardiovascular system circulates to tissues, while the digestive system provides nutrients needed for energy and repair.

Coordination among these systems ensures homeostasis, the maintenance of a stable internal environment despite external changes. This integrated approach allows the body to respond to stimuli, repair damage, and adapt to varying conditions. For example, when you exercise, your muscles require more oxygen and nutrients, which increases your heart rate and breathing rate. Your digestive system also adjusts by absorbing more nutrients from food. This seamless integration among systems is critical for overall health and survival.

Each system contributes to the body's functionality in a unique way. The cardiovascular system circulates blood, delivering oxygen and nutrients while removing waste products. The respiratory system ensures a continuous supply of oxygen and the removal of carbon dioxide. The digestive system breaks down food into absorbable nutrients. The nervous system processes sensory information and directs responses. The musculoskeletal system enables movement and support. The immune system defends against pathogens. The endocrine system regulates bodily functions through hormones. The urinary system manages waste and maintains fluid balance. The reproductive system ensures the continuation of species. Together, these systems create a resilient, adaptable organism capable of surviving in diverse environments.

The cardiovascular system, also known as the circulatory system, comprises the heart, blood vessels, and blood. Its primary function is to transport oxygen, nutrients, hormones, and waste products throughout the body. The heart, a muscular organ, acts as the pump, propelling blood through a network of arteries, veins, and capillaries.

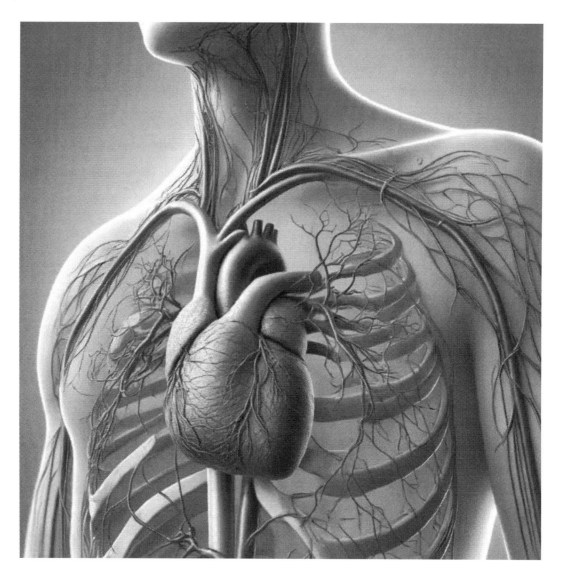

Blood flow follows a double circulation pathway: systemic and pulmonary circulation. In systemic circulation, oxygenated blood from the left ventricle is distributed to body tissues through the aorta and returned deoxygenated to the right atrium via veins. In pulmonary circulation, deoxygenated blood from the right ventricle is sent to the lungs through the pulmonary arteries, where it gets oxygenated and returned to the left atrium via pulmonary veins.

Arteries carry oxygen-rich blood away from the heart, while veins carry oxygen-depleted blood back to the heart. Capillaries, tiny blood vessels, facilitate the exchange of oxygen, nutrients, and waste between blood and tissues. The walls of capillaries are thin enough to allow the exchange of gases, nutrients, and waste products between blood and body tissues. This efficient exchange system ensures that all cells receive the nutrients they need and can dispose of their waste products.

Blood consists of red blood cells, white blood cells, platelets, and plasma. Red blood cells transport oxygen using hemoglobin, white blood cells defend against infections, platelets aid in clotting, and plasma, the liquid component, carries various substances throughout the body. This complex composition allows blood to perform its multiple roles, from delivering essential nutrients to fighting infections and repairing damage.

The heart's structure is uniquely designed for its function. It has four chambers: two atria and two ventricles. The atria receive blood entering the heart, while the ventricles pump blood out. Valves between the chambers ensure unidirectional blood flow, preventing backflow and maintaining efficient circulation. The heart's electrical conduction system coordinates the heartbeat, ensuring the chambers contract in a synchronized manner to effectively pump blood. Regular exercise, a balanced diet, and avoiding risk factors like smoking and excessive alcohol consumption are vital for maintaining cardiovascular health.

Breathing Easy: The Respiratory System

The respiratory system is responsible for gas exchange, supplying oxygen to the body and removing carbon dioxide. It consists of the nasal cavity, pharynx, larynx, trachea, bronchi, and lungs. Air enters through the nasal cavity, where it is filtered, warmed, and humidified. It then passes through the pharynx and larynx into the trachea, which branches into bronchi leading to the lungs.

Within the lungs, bronchi further divide into smaller bronchioles ending in alveoli, tiny air sacs where gas exchange occurs. Oxygen diffuses from alveoli into the blood, and carbon dioxide diffuses from the blood into alveoli to be exhaled. The alveoli provide a large surface area, ensuring efficient gas exchange. Surfactant, a substance coating the alveoli, prevents them from collapsing and reduces the work of breathing.

The diaphragm and intercostal muscles play crucial roles in ventilation, expanding and contracting the thoracic cavity to facilitate breathing. During inhalation, the diaphragm contracts and moves downward, enlarging the chest cavity and reducing pressure, drawing air into the lungs. During exhalation, the diaphragm relaxes and moves upward, compressing the chest cavity and expelling air from the lungs.

Respiratory control centers in the brainstem regulate breathing rate and depth, ensuring adequate oxygen intake and carbon dioxide removal to maintain blood pH and homeostasis. Chemoreceptors in the blood vessels monitor levels of oxygen and carbon dioxide, sending signals to the brain to adjust breathing as needed. This automatic regulation ensures that the body's oxygen needs are met, even during varying levels of physical activity.

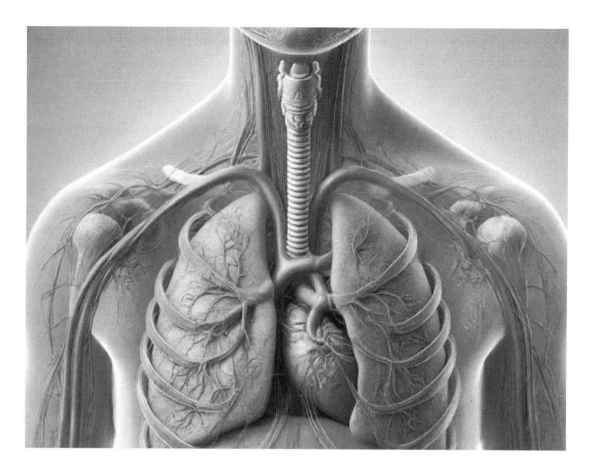

Proper respiratory function is vital for overall health. Conditions such as asthma, chronic obstructive pulmonary disease (COPD), and pneumonia can impair breathing, reducing oxygen delivery to tissues and causing significant health issues. Preventative measures, including avoiding smoking, reducing exposure to pollutants, and maintaining a healthy lifestyle, can support respiratory health and prevent diseases.

Digestive System: Fueling the Body

The digestive system breaks down food into nutrients the body can absorb and use for energy, growth, and repair. It consists of the gastrointestinal (GI) tract and accessory organs like the liver, pancreas, and gallbladder. The GI tract includes the mouth, esophagus, stomach, small intestine, and large intestine.

Digestion begins in the mouth, where chewing and saliva break down food. Saliva contains enzymes like amylase that start digesting carbohydrates. The esophagus transports food to the stomach through peristaltic movements. In the stomach, gastric juices containing hydrochloric acid and pepsin further digest proteins. The stomach's muscular walls churn food, turning it into a semi-liquid mixture called chyme.

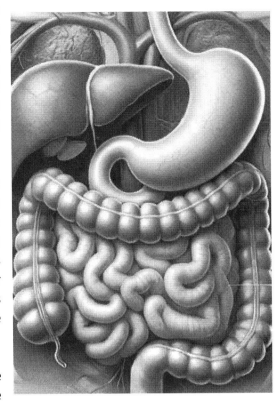

Chyme moves into the small intestine, where most nutrient absorption occurs. The small intestine is divided into three sections: the duodenum, jejunum, and ileum. Enzymes from the pancreas and bile from the liver aid in breaking down proteins, carbohydrates, and fats. The small intestine's lining, with villi and microvilli, increases the surface area for nutrient absorption into the bloodstream. Each villus contains blood vessels and a lymphatic vessel, facilitating the transport of absorbed nutrients.

The large intestine absorbs water and forms feces, which are excreted through the rectum and anus. The large intestine also hosts beneficial bacteria that produce vitamins and aid in digestion. This microbiome plays a crucial role in maintaining digestive health and overall well-being.

Proper digestion is essential for maintaining energy levels and overall health. Issues such as acid reflux, irritable bowel syndrome (IBS), and celiac disease can disrupt digestion, leading to discomfort and nutritional deficiencies. A balanced diet rich in fiber, adequate hydration, and regular physical activity support healthy digestion and prevent digestive disorders.

Nervous System: The Body's Command Center

The nervous system controls and coordinates body activities by transmitting electrical signals. It consists of the central nervous system (CNS) and peripheral nervous system (PNS). The CNS, comprising the brain and spinal cord, processes information and sends instructions. The PNS, consisting of nerves, connects the CNS to the rest of the body.

Neurons, the functional units of the nervous system, transmit signals through electrical impulses. A neuron has a cell body, dendrites that receive signals, and an axon that sends signals. Synapses are junctions where neurons communicate with other neurons, muscles, or glands through neurotransmitters. These chemical messengers bridge the gap between neurons, allowing the transmission of signals across the synaptic cleft.

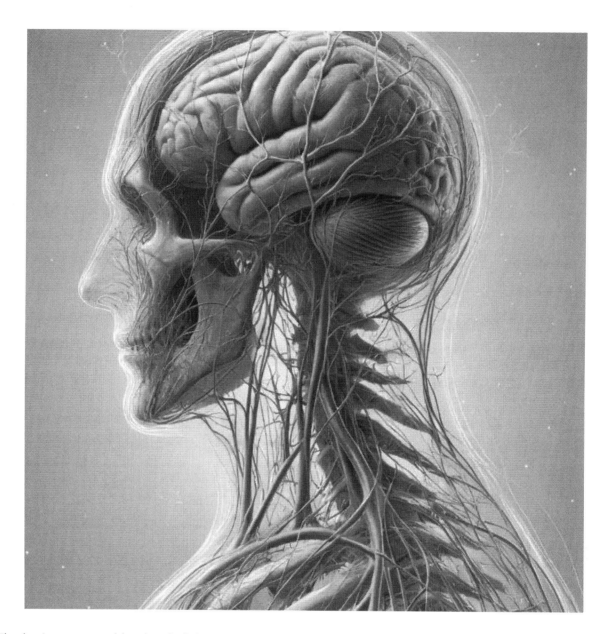

The brain, protected by the skull, has regions responsible for different functions, including the cerebrum (thought and memory), cerebellum (coordination), and brainstem (basic life functions). The cerebrum is divided into hemispheres and lobes, each associated with specific functions such as sensory perception, motor control, and cognitive abilities. The cerebellum coordinates voluntary movements and balance, while the brainstem regulates vital functions like heart rate and breathing.

The spinal cord, encased in the vertebral column, transmits signals between the brain and body. It also houses reflex arcs, which allow for rapid, involuntary responses to stimuli. Reflexes protect the body from harm by enabling quick reactions to potential dangers, such as pulling a hand away from a hot surface.

The autonomic nervous system, a part of the PNS, controls involuntary functions like heart rate and digestion, further divided into the sympathetic (fight or flight) and parasympathetic (rest and digest) systems. The sympathetic system prepares the body for action, increasing heart rate and diverting blood to muscles, while the parasympathetic system promotes relaxation and recovery.

Maintaining a healthy nervous system is crucial for overall well-being. Regular mental and physical exercise, a balanced diet, adequate sleep, and stress management are essential for supporting nervous system function and preventing disorders such as Alzheimer's disease, multiple sclerosis, and neuropathy.

Musculoskeletal System: Movement Mechanics

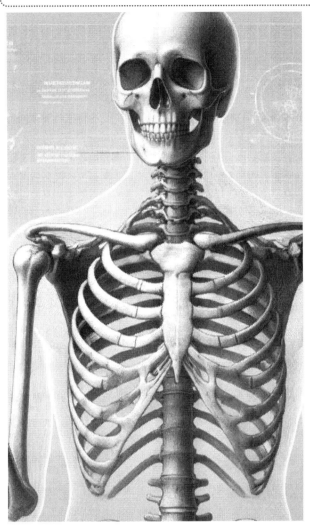

The musculoskeletal system provides structure, support, and the ability to move. It consists of bones, muscles, joints, cartilage, and ligaments. Bones form the skeleton, providing a framework and protecting vital organs. Muscles, attached to bones by tendons, contract to produce movement. Joints, where bones meet, allow for various types of movement, and cartilage reduces friction and absorbs shock.

There are 206 bones in the adult human body, categorized into the axial skeleton (skull, vertebral column, and rib cage) and the appendicular skeleton (limbs and girdles). Bones are dynamic, constantly being remodeled by osteoblasts (bone-forming cells) and osteoclasts (bone-resorbing cells). This remodeling process allows bones to adapt to stress and repair themselves after injuries.

Muscles are classified into skeletal (voluntary), cardiac (heart), and smooth (involuntary) muscles. Skeletal muscles work in pairs; when one contracts, the other relaxes, facilitating movement. Muscle contractions are controlled by motor neurons, which release neurotransmitters at neuromuscular junctions. The coordination between the nervous and muscular systems ensures smooth, precise movements.

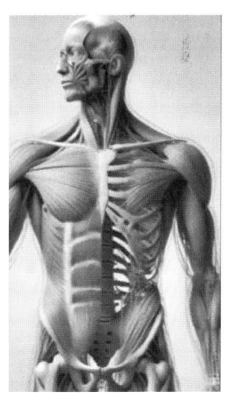

Ligaments connect bones at joints, providing stability, while tendons attach muscles to bones, enabling movement. Joints come in various types, such as hinge joints (elbows and knees) allowing movement in one direction, and ball-and-socket joints (shoulders and hips) allowing rotational movement. Cartilage cushions joints, reducing friction and preventing bone wear.

Proper nutrition, regular exercise, and avoiding injuries are crucial for maintaining musculoskeletal health. Conditions like osteoporosis, arthritis, and muscular dystrophy can impair the function of the musculoskeletal system, leading to pain and limited mobility. Weight-bearing exercises, a diet rich in calcium and vitamin D, and proper body mechanics can help prevent these conditions and promote long-term musculoskeletal health.

Immune System: Defending the Body

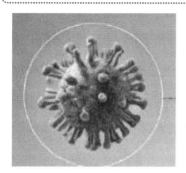

The immune system protects the body from infections and diseases. It consists of innate (nonspecific) and adaptive (specific) immunity. The innate immune system is the body's first line of defense, including physical barriers (skin and mucous membranes), phagocytic cells, natural killer cells, and inflammatory responses.

The adaptive immune system provides a targeted response to specific pathogens. It involves lymphocytes, including B cells and T cells. B cells produce antibodies that neutralize pathogens, while T cells destroy infected cells and coordinate the immune response. The adaptive immune system has memory, enabling a faster and more effective response to subsequent infections by the same pathogen.

The skin and mucous membranes act as physical barriers, preventing pathogens from entering the body. If pathogens breach these barriers, phagocytic cells like macrophages and neutrophils engulf and destroy them. Natural killer cells target and kill infected or cancerous cells, while the inflammatory response recruits immune cells to the site of infection or injury, promoting healing and preventing the spread of infection.

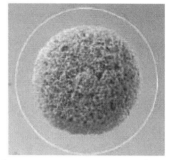

The lymphatic system supports the immune system by transporting lymph, a fluid containing immune cells, throughout the body. Lymph nodes, scattered along the lymphatic vessels, filter lymph and trap pathogens. The spleen and thymus are also important immune organs, with the spleen filtering blood and removing old or damaged red blood cells, and the thymus maturing T cells.

Vaccination is a critical tool in preventing infectious diseases by training the adaptive immune system to recognize and respond to specific pathogens. Maintaining a healthy immune system involves a balanced diet, regular exercise, adequate sleep, and stress management. Avoiding excessive use of antibiotics, which can disrupt the microbiome and promote antibiotic resistance, is also important.

Endocrine System: Hormonal Harmony

The endocrine system regulates bodily functions through hormones, chemical messengers released into the bloodstream by glands. Major endocrine glands include the pituitary, thyroid, parathyroid, adrenal, and pineal glands, as well as the pancreas, ovaries, and testes. Each gland produces specific hormones that regulate various processes, such as growth, metabolism, and reproduction.

The pituitary gland, often called the "master gland," controls other endocrine glands and releases hormones like growth hormone (GH), thyroid-stimulating hormone (TSH), and adrenocorticotropic hormone (ACTH). The hypothalamus, located above the pituitary, regulates its function by releasing hormones that stimulate or inhibit pituitary hormone production.

The thyroid gland produces thyroid hormones (T3 and T4), which regulate metabolism, energy levels, and growth. The parathyroid glands

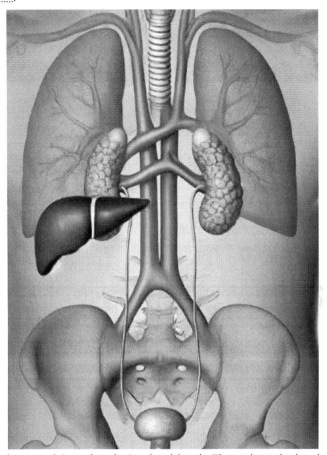

produce parathyroid hormone (PTH), which regulates calcium levels in the blood. The adrenal glands produce hormones like cortisol, which helps the body respond to stress, and aldosterone, which regulates blood pressure and electrolyte balance.

The pancreas produces insulin and glucagon, hormones that regulate blood sugar levels. Insulin lowers blood sugar by promoting glucose uptake into cells, while glucagon raises blood sugar by stimulating the release of glucose from the liver. The ovaries produce estrogen and progesterone, regulating the menstrual cycle and supporting pregnancy, while the testes produce testosterone, regulating sperm production and male secondary sexual characteristics.

Hormonal imbalances can lead to various disorders, such as diabetes, hypothyroidism, and Cushing's syndrome. Managing these conditions often involves medication, lifestyle changes, and regular monitoring. A healthy diet, regular exercise, and stress management can support endocrine health and prevent hormonal imbalances.

Urinary System: Waste Management

The urinary system removes waste products from the blood and maintains fluid and electrolyte balance. It consists of the kidneys, ureters, bladder, and urethra. The kidneys filter blood, removing waste products and excess substances, which form urine. This filtration process occurs in nephrons, the functional units of the kidneys.

Each kidney contains approximately one million nephrons, each consisting of a glomerulus and a renal tubule. Blood enters the glomerulus, where filtration occurs, and the filtrate passes through the renal tubule, where reabsorption and secretion modify its composition. Essential substances like water, glucose, and electrolytes are reabsorbed into the bloodstream, while waste products and excess substances are excreted as urine.

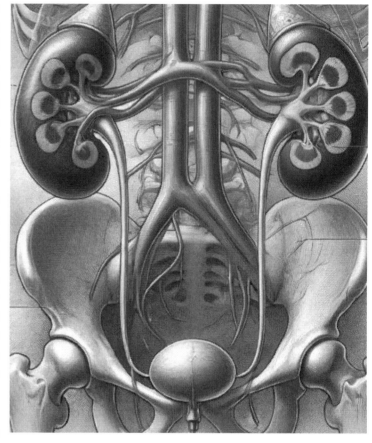

Urine flows from the kidneys through the ureters to the bladder, where it is stored until excretion through the urethra. The bladder's muscular walls stretch to accommodate increasing volumes of urine and contract during urination to expel urine. The process of urination is controlled by both voluntary and involuntary muscles, ensuring efficient and timely elimination of waste.

The urinary system also plays a crucial role in regulating blood pressure, red blood cell production, and acid-base balance. The kidneys produce renin, an enzyme that regulates blood pressure, and erythropoietin, a hormone that stimulates red blood cell production. They also maintain acid-base balance by excreting hydrogen ions and reabsorbing bicarbonate.

Maintaining urinary health involves staying hydrated, practicing good hygiene, and managing conditions like diabetes and hypertension that can affect kidney function. Conditions such as urinary tract infections (UTIs), kidney stones, and chronic kidney disease can impair the urinary system's function, leading to serious health issues. Early detection and treatment of these conditions are essential for preserving kidney health and overall well-being.

Reproductive System: The Circle of Life

The reproductive system ensures the continuation of the species through the production of offspring. It involves the production, maturation, and union of gametes (sperm and eggs), as well as the development and birth of a new organism. The male reproductive system includes the testes, vas deferens, prostate gland, and penis, while the female reproductive system includes the ovaries, fallopian tubes, uterus, and vagina.

In males, the testes produce sperm and testosterone, the hormone responsible for male secondary sexual characteristics and sperm production. Sperm mature in the epididymis and travel through the vas deferens during ejaculation. The prostate gland and seminal vesicles add fluids to sperm, forming semen, which is expelled through the penis.

In females, the ovaries produce eggs (ova) and hormones like estrogen and progesterone, which regulate the menstrual cycle and support pregnancy. During ovulation, an egg is released from an ovary and travels through the fallopian tube, where fertilization by a sperm can occur. The fertilized egg (zygote) implants in the uterus, where it develops into an embryo and eventually a fetus. The uterus provides nourishment and protection to the developing fetus until birth.

The menstrual cycle prepares the female body for pregnancy each month, involving the growth and shedding of the uterine lining. If fertilization does not occur, the lining is shed during menstruation. Hormonal regulation ensures the coordination of ovulation and the menstrual cycle.

Reproductive health is essential for fertility and overall well-being. Conditions such as polycystic ovary syndrome (PCOS), endometriosis, and infertility can affect reproductive function. Regular medical check-ups, a healthy lifestyle, and safe sexual practices support reproductive health and prevent complications.

Homeostasis: Maintaining Balance

Homeostasis is the maintenance of a stable internal environment despite external changes. It involves the regulation of factors like temperature, pH, and fluid balance, ensuring optimal conditions for cellular function. Various systems in the body work together to achieve homeostasis, responding to changes through feedback mechanisms.

Negative feedback mechanisms are the most common, where a change in a factor triggers a response that counteracts the change, restoring balance. For example, if body temperature rises, the hypothalamus triggers sweating and vasodilation to cool the body. If blood sugar levels rise, the pancreas releases insulin to promote glucose uptake by cells, lowering blood sugar levels.

Positive feedback mechanisms amplify a change, driving processes to completion. An example is childbirth, where the release of oxytocin intensifies uterine contractions, accelerating labor until delivery occurs. While less common, positive feedback is crucial in specific scenarios requiring rapid completion of a process.

The endocrine and nervous systems play central roles in regulating homeostasis. Hormones and neurotransmitters act as messengers, coordinating responses to maintain balance. The kidneys regulate fluid and electrolyte balance, while the liver processes nutrients and detoxifies substances. The respiratory system maintains oxygen and carbon dioxide levels, while the cardiovascular system distributes resources and removes waste.

Homeostasis is vital for health and survival. Disruptions can lead to conditions like dehydration, acidosis, and hypothermia. Chronic diseases, infections, and environmental factors can challenge the body's ability to maintain homeostasis. Supporting homeostasis involves a balanced diet, regular exercise, adequate hydration, and avoiding harmful substances. Understanding and supporting the body's regulatory mechanisms promote resilience and well-being.

Life sciences encompass a vast array of disciplines focused on the study of living organisms and their interactions with the environment. From the microscopic intricacies of cellular processes to the broad dynamics of ecosystems, life sciences seek to understand the fundamental principles that govern life on Earth. This chapter delves into some of the core topics within life sciences, including the blueprint of life encoded in DNA and genetics, the complex processes that sustain cellular functions, the mechanisms of cell division, the intricate webs of ecosystems and environments, the principles of evolution and natural selection, and the profound impact of human activities on our planet. By exploring these subjects, we gain a deeper appreciation of the diversity of life and the interconnectedness of all living things.

DNA and Genetics: The Blueprint of Life

Deoxyribonucleic acid (DNA) is the hereditary material in all known living organisms and many viruses. It carries the genetic instructions used in the growth, development, functioning, and reproduction of all living things. The structure of DNA is a double helix, composed of two strands twisted around each other. Each strand is made up of nucleotides, which include a sugar, a phosphate group, and a nitrogenous base. The sequence of these bases (adenine, thymine, cytosine, and guanine) encodes genetic information.

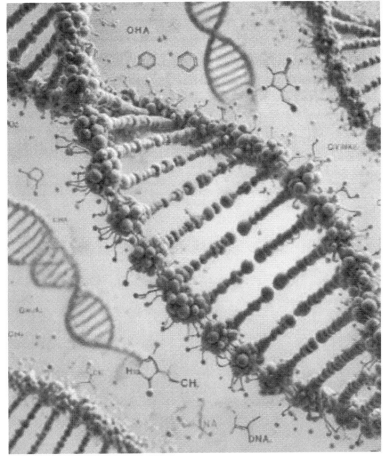

Genes, segments of DNA, are the fundamental units of heredity. They dictate the synthesis of proteins, which perform a wide array of functions within organisms. Proteins are synthesized through two key processes: transcription and translation. During transcription, a gene's DNA sequence is copied into messenger RNA (mRNA). This mRNA then travels from the nucleus to the cytoplasm, where it is translated by ribosomes to form proteins. The specific sequence of amino acids in a protein determines its structure and function.

Genetic variation arises from mutations, changes in the DNA sequence. Mutations can be caused by errors during DNA replication, exposure to mutagens, or viral infections. While many mutations are neutral or harmful, some can be beneficial and contribute to an organism's adaptability and evolution.

Inheritance patterns are governed by Mendelian genetics, which describes how traits are passed from parents to offspring through dominant and recessive alleles. However, many traits are influenced by multiple genes (polygenic inheritance) and environmental factors. Understanding genetics enables us to comprehend how traits are inherited, how genetic disorders arise, and how genetic technologies can be applied in medicine and agriculture.

The study of genetics has led to significant advancements in biotechnology, such as gene editing and genetic engineering. Techniques like CRISPR-Cas9 allow for precise modification of DNA sequences, offering potential treatments for genetic disorders and the development of genetically modified organisms (GMOs) with desirable traits. These advancements have far-reaching implications, from curing genetic diseases to enhancing agricultural productivity.

Genetic research also plays a crucial role in personalized medicine, an emerging field that tailors medical treatment to individual genetic profiles. By understanding a patient's genetic makeup, doctors can predict responses to drugs, identify risk factors for diseases, and develop targeted therapies. This approach promises to improve the efficacy of treatments and reduce adverse effects.

Understanding Cellular Processes and Functions

Cells, the basic units of life, perform a myriad of processes essential for survival and function. These processes include metabolism, cellular respiration, protein synthesis, and signal transduction, each involving intricate biochemical pathways and molecular interactions.

Metabolism encompasses all chemical reactions within a cell, divided into catabolism (breaking down molecules for energy) and anabolism (synthesizing complex molecules from simpler ones). ATP (adenosine triphosphate) serves as the primary energy currency in cells, fueling various metabolic reactions. Enzymes play a crucial role in metabolism by lowering the activation energy of reactions, thereby increasing their rate.

Cellular respiration is a catabolic process that converts glucose and oxygen into ATP, carbon dioxide, and water. It consists of glycolysis, the citric acid cycle, and oxidative phosphorylation. Glycolysis occurs in the cytoplasm, breaking glucose into pyruvate while generating a small amount of ATP. Pyruvate enters the mitochondria, where the citric acid cycle produces electron carriers that transfer energy to the electron transport chain. Oxidative phosphorylation, occurring in the inner mitochondrial membrane, generates the bulk of ATP through chemiosmosis.

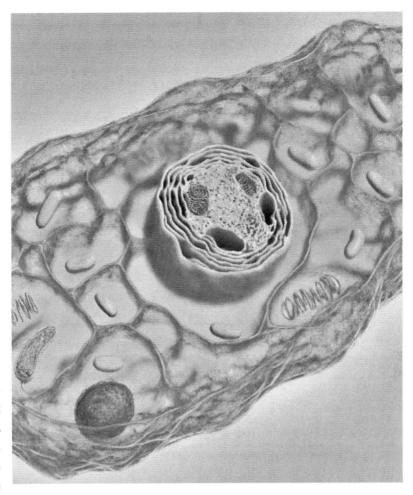

Protein synthesis, essential for cell function and growth, involves transcription and translation. During transcription, a gene's DNA sequence is transcribed into mRNA, which exits the nucleus and is translated by ribosomes into a polypeptide chain. The sequence of amino acids in the polypeptide determines its folding and function as a protein. Post-translational modifications, such as phosphorylation and glycosylation, further refine protein function and localization.

Signal transduction pathways enable cells to respond to external stimuli and communicate with each other. These pathways often involve receptor proteins on the cell surface that bind to signaling molecules (ligands). This binding triggers a cascade of intracellular events, activating or inhibiting specific cellular functions. For example, the insulin signaling pathway regulates glucose uptake and metabolism in response to blood sugar levels. Dysregulation of signal transduction pathways can lead to diseases such as cancer and diabetes.

Cellular processes are tightly regulated to maintain homeostasis and respond to changes in the environment. Feedback mechanisms, such as negative feedback loops, ensure that cellular functions remain within optimal ranges. Disruptions in these processes can lead to diseases such as cancer, diabetes, and neurodegenerative disorders. Research in cell biology continues to uncover the mechanisms underlying these processes, leading to new therapeutic strategies.

The Magic of Cell Division: Mitosis and Meiosis

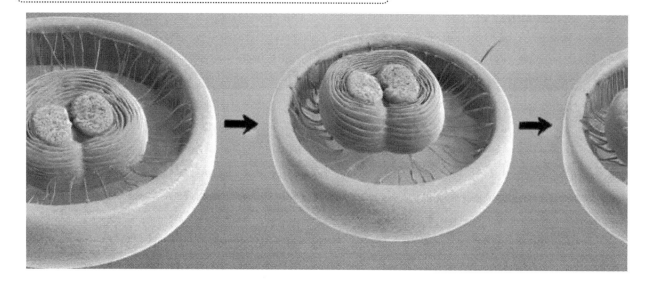

Cell division is a fundamental process by which cells replicate and pass on genetic information. There are two main types of cell division: mitosis and meiosis. Mitosis results in two genetically identical daughter cells, while meiosis produces four genetically diverse gametes (sperm or eggs).

Mitosis is essential for growth, tissue repair, and asexual reproduction. It consists of several phases: prophase, metaphase, anaphase, telophase, and cytokinesis. During prophase, chromatin condenses into visible chromosomes, and the mitotic spindle forms. In metaphase, chromosomes align at the cell's equator. Anaphase follows, with sister chromatids separating and moving to opposite poles. Telophase involves the reformation of the nuclear envelope around the separated chromatids, now individual chromosomes. Finally, cytokinesis divides the cytoplasm, resulting in two daughter cells.

Meiosis, on the other hand, reduces the chromosome number by half, producing haploid cells from a diploid parent cell. This reduction is crucial for sexual reproduction, ensuring offspring have the correct chromosome number. Meiosis consists of two divisions: meiosis I and meiosis II. Meiosis I separates homologous chromosomes, and meiosis II separates sister chromatids, similar to mitosis. Genetic recombination, occurring during prophase I through crossing over, increases genetic diversity by exchanging DNA between homologous chromosomes.

Errors in cell division can lead to genetic disorders and diseases. For instance, nondisjunction, the failure of chromosomes to separate properly, can result in conditions like Down syndrome, where an individual has an extra copy of chromosome 21. Additionally, mutations arising during cell division can lead to cancer if they affect genes that control cell growth and division.

Understanding the mechanisms of cell division provides insights into developmental biology, cancer, and genetic disorders. Research continues to explore the regulation of these processes, aiming to develop targeted therapies for diseases caused by cell division abnormalities. Advances in technologies such as CRISPR and live-cell imaging are enhancing our ability to study and manipulate cell division with unprecedented precision.

Ecosystems and Environments: Interconnected Webs

Ecosystems are complex networks of living organisms interacting with their physical environment. They encompass biotic components (plants, animals, microorganisms) and abiotic components (water, soil, air, nutrients). These interactions create a dynamic balance, sustaining life and driving ecological processes.

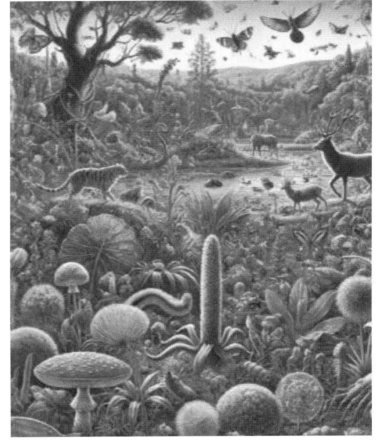

Ecosystems vary in scale and complexity, from small ponds to vast forests and oceans. Each ecosystem has a unique structure and function, influenced by factors such as climate, geography, and human activities. Primary productivity, the rate at which plants and other autotrophs convert solar energy into biomass, forms the foundation of ecosystem energy flow.

Food webs depict the transfer of energy and nutrients through trophic levels, from primary producers (plants) to primary consumers (herbivores), secondary consumers (carnivores), and decomposers. These interactions maintain ecosystem stability and resilience, enabling organisms to adapt to changes and disturbances.

Biogeochemical cycles, such as the carbon, nitrogen, and water cycles, regulate the flow of essential elements through ecosystems. These cycles involve processes like photosynthesis, respiration, decomposition, and nutrient uptake, ensuring the availability of resources for living organisms. Disruptions in these cycles, often caused by human activities, can lead to environmental issues such as climate change, eutrophication, and pollution.

Biodiversity, the variety of life forms within an ecosystem, enhances its stability and resilience. Diverse ecosystems are more productive and better able to withstand environmental changes and disturbances. Conservation efforts aim to protect biodiversity by preserving habitats, restoring degraded ecosystems, and mitigating human impacts.

Ecosystems provide vital services to humans, including food, clean water, air purification, climate regulation, and recreational opportunities. Recognizing the interconnectedness of ecosystems and human well-being is essential for sustainable development and environmental stewardship.

Evolution is the process by which populations of organisms change over time through variations in their genetic makeup. Natural selection, a key mechanism of evolution, was first described by Charles Darwin. It explains how traits that enhance an organism's survival and reproduction become more common in a population over generations.

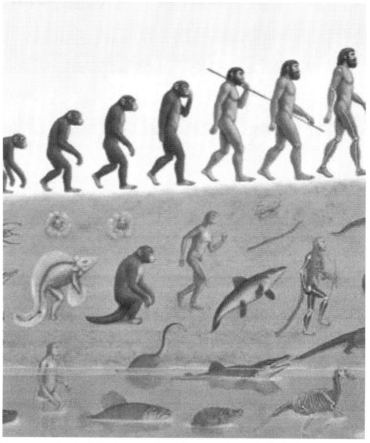

Natural selection operates on genetic variation within a population. Variations arise from mutations, genetic recombination, and gene flow. Individuals with advantageous traits are more likely to survive and reproduce, passing these traits to their offspring. Over time, these traits become more prevalent, leading to the adaptation of populations to their environments.

Evolutionary processes also include genetic drift, gene flow, and sexual selection. Genetic drift is the random fluctuation of allele frequencies in a population, particularly in small populations. Gene flow, the movement of genes between populations, can introduce new genetic material and increase genetic diversity. Sexual selection, a form of natural selection, involves traits that enhance mating success, such as elaborate displays or behaviors.

Speciation, the formation of new species, occurs when populations become reproductively isolated and diverge genetically. This can result from geographic isolation, ecological differences, or behavioral changes. Over long periods, these processes generate the vast diversity of life observed today.

The evidence for evolution is abundant, including the fossil record, comparative anatomy, molecular biology, and biogeography. Fossils provide a historical record of life, showing the progression of forms over time. Comparative anatomy reveals similarities in the structures of different organisms, suggesting common ancestry. Molecular biology examines genetic similarities and differences, supporting evolutionary relationships. Biogeography studies the distribution of species, revealing patterns consistent with evolutionary processes.

Understanding evolution provides insights into the origins of biodiversity, the adaptation of organisms to their environments, and the processes driving biological change. It also informs fields such as medicine, agriculture, and conservation, helping to address challenges like antibiotic resistance, crop improvement, and species conservation.

Human Impact on Our Planet

Human activities have profoundly impacted the planet, altering ecosystems, climate, and biodiversity. The rapid growth of the human population, coupled with industrialization, urbanization, and resource exploitation, has led to significant environmental changes.

Deforestation, the clearing of forests for agriculture, logging, and development, reduces biodiversity, disrupts ecosystems, and contributes to climate change by releasing stored carbon dioxide. Forests play a critical role in regulating the climate, cycling nutrients, and providing habitats for countless species. Preserving and restoring forests is essential for maintaining ecological balance and mitigating climate change.

Pollution, including air, water, and soil pollution, poses serious threats to human health and the environment. Industrial emissions, vehicle exhaust, agricultural runoff, and plastic waste contaminate natural resources, harm wildlife, and disrupt ecosystems. Reducing pollution through cleaner technologies, sustainable practices, and regulatory measures is crucial for protecting the planet.

Climate change, driven by greenhouse gas emissions from burning fossil fuels, deforestation, and industrial processes, is causing global temperatures to rise, leading to more frequent and severe weather events, melting ice caps, rising sea levels, and shifting ecosystems. Mitigating climate change requires reducing emissions, transitioning to renewable energy sources, and enhancing carbon sinks.

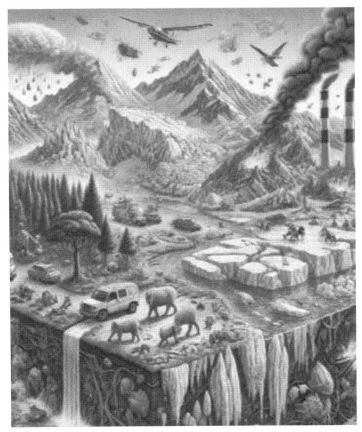

Overfishing and habitat destruction threaten marine ecosystems, reducing fish populations, altering food webs, and degrading coral reefs and other critical habitats. Sustainable fishing practices, marine protected areas, and habitat restoration efforts are essential for preserving ocean health and biodiversity.

Urbanization and infrastructure development fragment habitats, reduce green spaces, and increase pollution and resource consumption. Sustainable urban planning, green infrastructure, and conservation of natural areas within cities can mitigate these impacts and enhance urban resilience.

Conservation efforts aim to protect endangered species, restore degraded habitats, and promote sustainable resource use. International agreements, such as the Convention on Biological Diversity and the Paris Agreement, provide frameworks for global cooperation on environmental issues. Local and community-based initiatives also play a vital role in conservation and sustainability.

Educating and engaging people about the importance of environmental stewardship and sustainable practices is essential for fostering a culture of conservation. Individuals can contribute by reducing their carbon footprint, supporting sustainable products, conserving resources, and participating in conservation efforts.

By recognizing and addressing the interconnected challenges of environmental degradation, climate change, and biodiversity loss, we can work towards a more sustainable and resilient future for our planet and all its inhabitants.

PHYSICAL SCIENCES AND CHEMISTRY

The physical sciences encompass a wide range of disciplines that explore the fundamental principles governing the natural world. From the behavior of subatomic particles to the dynamics of celestial bodies, physical sciences seek to understand the underlying laws of nature. This chapter delves into key topics within physical sciences and chemistry, including the nature of chemical reactions, the organization and significance of the periodic table, the distinctions between compounds and mixtures, the physics of everyday phenomena, the foundational laws of motion and energy, and the principles of waves and sound. By examining these subjects, we gain insight into the physical world and the scientific principles that shape our everyday experiences.

Chemical Reactions Demystified

Chemical reactions are processes in which substances, known as reactants, are transformed into different substances, called products. These reactions involve the breaking and forming of chemical bonds, leading to changes in the composition and properties of matter. Understanding chemical reactions is fundamental to the study of chemistry and has practical applications in various fields, including medicine, industry, and environmental science.

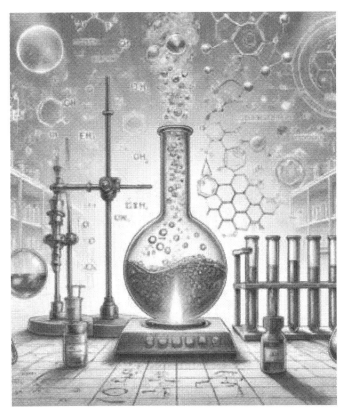

A chemical reaction can be represented by a chemical equation, which shows the reactants and products along with their respective quantities. For example, the combustion of methane (CH_4) in oxygen (O_2) can be represented as:

In this reaction, methane and oxygen react to form carbon dioxide (CO_2) and water (H_2O). The coefficients in the equation indicate the proportions in which the substances react.

Chemical reactions can be classified into different types based on their characteristics. Some common types include:

- Synthesis Reactions: Two or more simple substances combine to form a more complex substance.
- Decomposition Reactions: A complex substance breaks down into simpler substances.
- Single Displacement Reactions: An element replaces another element in a compound.

- Double Displacement Reactions: The ions of two compounds exchange places to form two new compounds.
- Combustion Reactions: A substance reacts with oxygen, releasing energy in the form of heat and light.

The rate of a chemical reaction is influenced by factors such as temperature, concentration of reactants, surface area, and the presence of catalysts. Catalysts are substances that increase the reaction rate without being consumed in the reaction. They work by providing an alternative reaction pathway with a lower activation energy.

Understanding the principles of chemical reactions enables us to manipulate them for various purposes. In industrial chemistry, reactions are optimized to maximize product yield and minimize waste. In biochemistry, enzyme-catalyzed reactions are essential for metabolic processes in living organisms. In environmental science, reactions are studied to understand and mitigate pollution.

The Periodic Table: Elements and Their Properties

The periodic table is a systematic arrangement of elements based on their atomic number, electron configurations, and recurring chemical properties. Developed by Dmitri Mendeleev in the 19th century, the periodic table has become a fundamental tool in chemistry for predicting the behavior of elements and their compounds.

Elements in the periodic table are organized into rows called periods and columns called groups or families. Each element is represented by a symbol, its atomic number (number of protons), and its atomic mass. Elements in the same group have similar chemical properties because they have the same number of valence electrons, which are the electrons involved in chemical bonding.

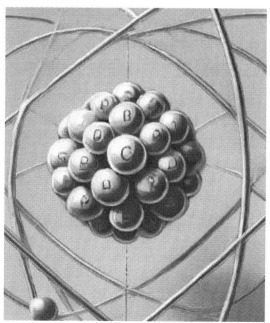

The periodic table is divided into several blocks based on the electron configuration of the elements:
- s-block: Includes groups 1 (alkali metals) and 2 (alkaline earth metals). These elements have their outermost electrons in s orbitals.
- p-block: Includes groups 13 to 18. Elements in this block have their outermost electrons in p orbitals.
- d-block: Includes transition metals, which have their outermost electrons in d orbitals.
- f-block: Includes lanthanides and actinides, which have their outermost electrons in f orbitals.

The periodic trends observed in the table include:

- Atomic Radius: Generally decreases across a period and increases down a group.
- Ionization Energy: The energy required to remove an electron from an atom. It generally increases across a period and decreases down a group.

- Electronegativity: A measure of an atom's ability to attract and hold electrons. It generally increases across a period and decreases down a group.
- Electron Affinity: The energy change when an electron is added to an atom. It generally becomes more negative across a period and varies less predictably down a group.

Understanding the periodic table allows chemists to predict the properties of elements and their compounds, facilitating the discovery of new materials and the development of chemical reactions. It also provides insights into the structure and behavior of atoms, which are the building blocks of matter.

Compounds and Mixtures Explained

Matter can be classified into pure substances and mixtures. Pure substances have a fixed composition and distinct properties. They can be either elements, which consist of only one type of atom, or compounds, which consist of two or more types of atoms chemically bonded together. Mixtures, on the other hand, are combinations of two or more substances that retain their individual properties and can be separated by physical means.

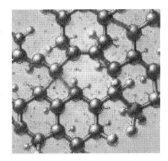

Compounds are substances formed when two or more elements chemically bond in fixed proportions. The properties of compounds are different from those of their constituent elements. For example, water (H_2O) is a compound composed of hydrogen and oxygen. While hydrogen is a flammable gas and oxygen supports combustion, water is a liquid that extinguishes fire. Compounds can be classified into different types based on the nature of their bonding:

- **Ionic Compounds**
  Formed by the transfer of electrons from one atom to another, resulting in the formation of positively charged ions (cations) and negatively charged ions (anions). These compounds typically have high melting and boiling points and conduct electricity when dissolved in water. Example: Sodium chloride (NaCl).

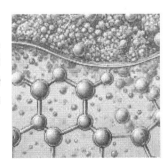

- **Covalent Compounds**
  Formed by the sharing of electrons between atoms. These compounds can exist as gases, liquids, or solids and have lower melting and boiling points compared to ionic compounds. They do not conduct electricity in the solid state. Example: Methane (CH_4).

- **Metallic Compounds**
  Consist of metal atoms bonded by a "sea" of delocalized electrons that are free to move throughout the structure. This type of bonding gives metals their characteristic properties, such as conductivity and malleability. Example: Iron (Fe).

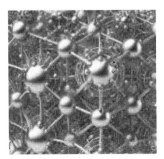

Mixtures are combinations of two or more substances that can be separated by physical means.

Mixtures can be homogeneous or heterogeneous

- **Homogeneous Mixtures (Solutions)**
  Have a uniform composition throughout. The components are evenly distributed, and the mixture appears as a single phase. Example: Saltwater.

- **Heterogeneous Mixtures**
  Have a non-uniform composition. The components are not evenly distributed, and distinct phases can be observed. Example: Sand and water.

Mixtures can be separated into their components using various physical methods, such as filtration, distillation, and chromatography. Understanding the differences between compounds and mixtures is essential for analyzing and manipulating materials in chemistry and related fields.

The Physics of Everyday Life

Physics is the study of matter, energy, and the fundamental forces of nature. It seeks to understand how the universe behaves, from the smallest particles to the largest structures. The principles of physics are evident in everyday life, explaining phenomena we encounter regularly.

- Mechanics, the branch of physics that deals with motion and forces, helps us understand how objects move and interact. For example, when riding a bicycle, we apply forces to the pedals, which are transmitted through the chain to the wheels, propelling the bicycle forward. The concepts of velocity, acceleration, and friction play crucial roles in this process.

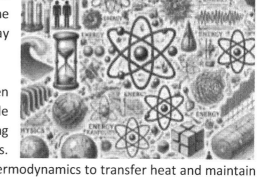

- Thermodynamics explores the relationships between heat, work, and energy. Everyday applications include cooking, where heat is transferred to food, causing chemical reactions that change its properties. Refrigerators and air conditioners use principles of thermodynamics to transfer heat and maintain desired temperatures.

- Electromagnetism studies electric and magnetic fields and their interactions. This branch of physics explains how electrical devices work, from light bulbs and motors to computers and smartphones. Electromagnetic waves, including visible light, radio waves, and microwaves, enable communication and information transfer in our daily lives.

- Optics focuses on the behavior of light. Understanding optics is essential for designing lenses, microscopes, telescopes, and other devices that manipulate light. Corrective eyewear, cameras, and fiber-optic communication systems rely on principles of optics to function effectively.

- Acoustics, the study of sound, explains how we hear and produce sounds. Musical instruments, speakers, and microphones operate based on acoustic principles. Understanding sound waves and their properties helps improve the quality of audio devices and design better acoustical environments in concert halls and recording studios.

- Nuclear Physics and Quantum Mechanics delve into the behavior of particles at the atomic and subatomic levels. These fields have led to advancements in medical imaging, such as MRI and PET scans, and the development of technologies like semiconductors and lasers.

Physics not only enhances our understanding of the natural world but also drives technological innovation, improving our quality of life and expanding our capabilities.

Laws of Motion and Energy

The laws of motion and energy are fundamental principles that describe how objects move and interact. These laws, formulated by Sir Isaac Newton and other physicists, provide the foundation for classical mechanics and have wide-ranging applications in science and engineering.

Newton's Laws of Motion describe the relationship between the motion of an object and the forces acting on it:

First Law

An object at rest stays at rest, and an object in motion continues in motion with a constant velocity unless acted upon by a net external force. This law explains why seat belts are essential in cars; without them, passengers would continue moving forward when the car suddenly stops.

Second Law

The acceleration of an object is directly proportional to the net force acting on it and inversely proportional to its mass. This can be expressed by the equation:
$$F = ma$$
where F is the net force, m is the mass, and a is the acceleration. This law is applied in various fields, from engineering to space travel, to determine the motion of objects under different forces.

Third Law

For every action, there is an equal and opposite reaction. This law explains phenomena such as a gun's recoil when fired and rockets' propulsion.

Energy is the ability to do work, and it exists in various forms, including kinetic, potential, thermal, electrical, and chemical energy. The Law of Conservation of Energy states that energy cannot be created or destroyed, only transformed from one form to another. This principle is observed in everyday activities, such as using a battery to power a flashlight, where chemical energy is converted into electrical energy and light and heat.

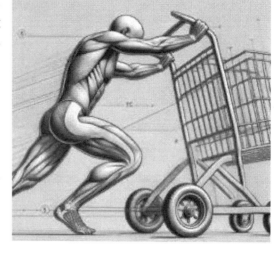

Work is done when a force acts on an object to move it a certain distance. The relationship between work, force, and distance is given by:

$$W = Fd$$

where W is the work done, F is the force applied, and d is the distance moved in the direction of the force.

Power is the rate at which work is done or energy is transferred. It is calculated as:

$$P = W/t$$

where P is the power, W is the work done, and t is the time taken. Understanding power is crucial in designing machines and engines that operate efficiently. These laws and principles provide the foundation for analyzing and predicting the behavior of physical systems, enabling the development of technologies and engineering solutions that improve our lives.

Waves and Sound: Understanding the Basics

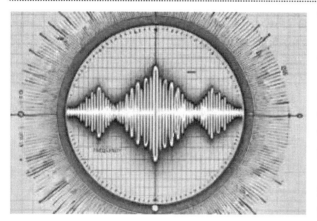

Waves are disturbances that transfer energy from one place to another without transferring matter. They can be classified into mechanical waves, which require a medium to travel through, and electromagnetic waves, which can travel through a vacuum. Mechanical waves include sound waves and water waves, while electromagnetic waves include light, radio waves, and X-rays.

Sound waves are longitudinal mechanical waves that travel through a medium, such as air, water, or solids. They are produced by vibrating objects and propagate by compressing and rarefying the medium. The speed of sound depends on the medium and its temperature; for example, sound travels faster in water than in air.

The properties of sound waves include frequency, wavelength, amplitude, and speed:

- Frequency is the number of wave cycles that pass a point per unit time, measured in hertz (Hz). It determines the pitch of the sound; higher frequencies produce higher pitches.
- Wavelength is the distance between two consecutive points in phase on a wave, such as from crest to crest or trough to trough.
- Amplitude is the maximum displacement of the wave from its equilibrium position, determining the loudness of the sound.

- Speed is the rate at which the wave propagates through the medium.

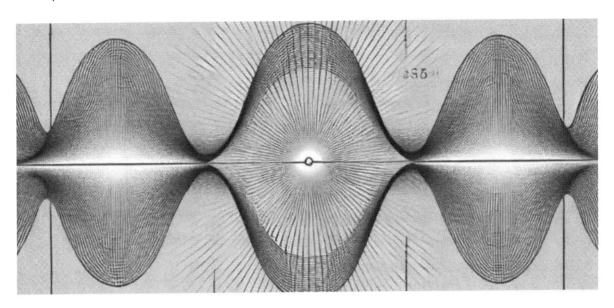

Electromagnetic waves are transverse waves that consist of oscillating electric and magnetic fields perpendicular to each other and the direction of propagation. They do not require a medium and can travel through the vacuum of space. The electromagnetic spectrum includes radio waves, microwaves, infrared, visible light, ultraviolet, X-rays, and gamma rays, each with different wavelengths and frequencies.

Understanding the principles of waves and sound is essential in various applications, from designing musical instruments and audio equipment to developing communication technologies and medical imaging techniques.

SCIENTIFIC INQUIRY AND METHOD

Scientific inquiry is the systematic investigation of natural phenomena through observation, experimentation, and analysis. It involves formulating questions, developing hypotheses, conducting experiments, and drawing conclusions based on empirical evidence. The scientific method is the cornerstone of this process, providing a structured approach to discovering new knowledge and validating or refuting existing theories. This chapter explores the key components of scientific inquiry and method, including the scientific method itself, conducting and analyzing experiments, drawing logical conclusions from studies, interpreting scientific literature, and the ethical considerations in scientific research. Through example scenarios, we will illustrate how these principles are applied in real-world scientific investigations.

The Scientific Method: Step-by-Step

The scientific method is a systematic approach used by scientists to investigate natural phenomena, acquire new knowledge, or correct and integrate previous knowledge. It is based on empirical and measurable evidence, subject to specific principles of reasoning. The scientific method involves several key steps:

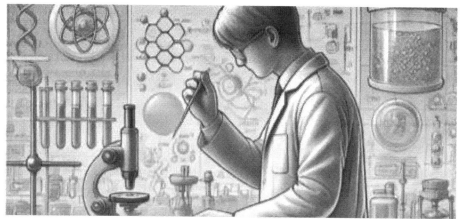

1. **Observation**

   This is the initial stage where a scientist makes an observation about a phenomenon or a set of data. Observations can come from previous research, natural occurrences, or unexpected events that spark curiosity. For example, a biologist might observe that a certain species of plant grows faster in one part of a forest than another, prompting further investigation.

2. **Question**

Based on the observation, a question is formulated. This question should be specific, measurable, and researchable. For instance, the biologist might ask, "How does the amount of sunlight affect the growth rate of this plant species?" This question is clear and directs the focus of the investigation.

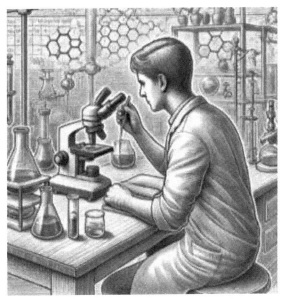

3. **Hypothesis**

A hypothesis is a tentative explanation or prediction that can be tested through experimentation. It is often structured as an "if-then" statement. For example, "If the amount of sunlight is increased, then the growth rate of the plant will also increase." This hypothesis provides a basis for designing experiments.

4. **Experiment**

This involves designing and conducting an experiment to test the hypothesis. The experiment must be controlled and repeatable, with independent variables (what you change), dependent variables (what you measure), and controlled variables (what you keep the same). In our example, the biologist might set up several plots of the plant species in different light conditions while keeping soil type and watering consistent.

5. **Data Collection**

During the experiment, data are meticulously recorded. This can involve quantitative data (numerical measurements) or qualitative data (descriptions or observations). Tools and techniques for data collection vary widely depending on the field of study but must be precise and accurate to ensure valid results. For instance, the biologist might measure the height of the plants weekly and record the number of leaves.

6. **Analysis**

Once the data are collected, they are analyzed to determine whether they support or refute the hypothesis. This can involve statistical analysis, graphing, and comparing results to the control group. The analysis helps to identify patterns, relationships, and potential anomalies in the data. For example, the biologist might use statistical software to compare the growth rates under different light conditions.

7. **Conclusion**

Based on the analysis, a conclusion is drawn. This conclusion should directly address the hypothesis, indicating whether it was supported or not. If the hypothesis is supported, the conclusion may lead to further questions and experiments. If it is not supported, the scientist may revise the hypothesis or develop new ones to test. For example, the biologist might conclude that increased sunlight does indeed lead to faster growth and might next investigate the optimal amount of sunlight.

8. **Communication**

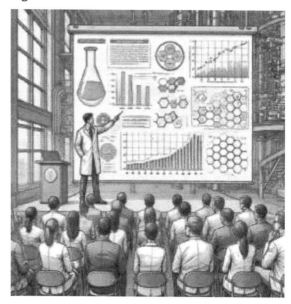

The final step is to communicate the results to the scientific community and the public. This can be done through research papers, presentations, or reports. Effective communication ensures that others can review, replicate, and build upon the findings. The biologist might publish the findings in a scientific journal or present them at a conference.

The scientific method is iterative, meaning that it often involves repeated cycles of hypothesis and experimentation, leading to increasingly refined knowledge and understanding.

Conducting and Analyzing Experiments

Conducting experiments is a fundamental part of the scientific method. It involves several key stages to ensure that the results are reliable and valid:

- **Planning**

  Before starting an experiment, detailed planning is crucial. This includes defining the research question, selecting the variables, and deciding on the experimental design. A well-planned experiment will have clear objectives, a detailed protocol, and a consideration of potential challenges. For example, if a chemist wants to test the effect of temperature on reaction rates, they must decide the temperature range, the reaction being studied, and how to measure the rate accurately.

- **Preparation**

  Gathering all necessary materials and equipment is the next step. This might involve sourcing chemicals, calibrating instruments, or preparing samples. Ensuring everything is ready and in working order before beginning the experiment helps to avoid delays and errors. For instance, the chemist might need to calibrate a thermometer and ensure all reagents are of high purity.

- **Execution**

  Conducting the experiment requires following the protocol precisely to ensure consistency and reliability. This includes carefully measuring and controlling variables, accurately recording data, and maintaining a clean and organized workspace. In the temperature experiment, the chemist would need to control the temperature precisely and measure reaction times consistently.

- **Data Collection**

  Data should be recorded in real-time and in a systematic manner. This may involve using data sheets, lab notebooks, or digital recording devices. Ensuring that data collection methods are consistent and precise is essential for subsequent analysis. The chemist might use a digital timer to record reaction times and enter these into a spreadsheet for analysis.

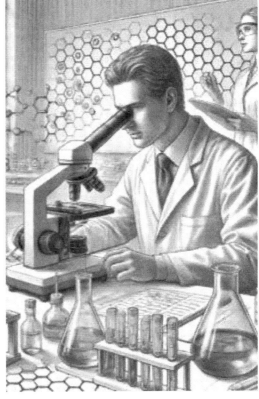

- **Analysis**

  Once the experiment is complete, the data are analyzed to identify trends and test the hypothesis. This often involves statistical analysis to determine the significance of the results. Tools such as spreadsheets, statistical software, and graphing tools can be used to analyze and visualize the data. The chemist might create graphs to show how reaction rates change with temperature and use statistical tests to confirm the significance of the findings.

- **Review and Repeat**

  Reviewing the results is critical. If the data do not support the hypothesis or if there are significant anomalies, the experiment may need to be repeated. Repetition helps to ensure that the results are reliable and not due to random chance or experimental error. The chemist might repeat the experiment multiple times to verify the consistency of the results.

Drawing Logical Conclusions from Studies

Drawing logical conclusions from studies involves interpreting the data and understanding its implications. Here are the steps to draw sound conclusions:

- **Summarize Findings**

  Begin by summarizing the main findings of the study. What do the data show? Identify key trends, differences, and patterns. For example, if a psychologist studies the effect of sleep on memory, they might find that participants who slept eight hours performed better on memory tests than those who slept four hours.

- **Compare with Hypothesis**

  Assess whether the findings support or refute the initial hypothesis. This comparison helps to determine the validity of the hypothesis. The psychologist would compare the performance of different sleep groups to the hypothesis that more sleep improves memory.

- **Consider Limitations**

  Every study has limitations, whether due to sample size, methodology, or external factors. Recognizing these limitations is important for understanding the scope and applicability of the conclusions. The psychologist might note that the study only

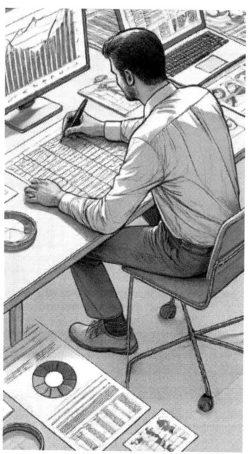

included college students, which limits the generalizability of the findings to other populations.

- **Contextualize Results**

  Place the findings within the broader context of existing research. How do the results align with or differ from previous studies? This helps to understand the significance and impact of the findings. The psychologist might reference other studies that have shown similar results or highlight differences that could be due to methodological variations.

- **Make Inferences**

  Based on the findings and their context, make logical inferences. What do the results imply about the phenomenon being studied? These inferences should be grounded in the data and not based on assumptions or speculation. The psychologist might infer that adequate sleep is crucial for optimal memory function and suggest practical applications for improving sleep hygiene.

- **Suggest Future Research**

  Identify areas for further study. What questions remain unanswered? How can future research build on these findings? Suggesting future research directions is a key part of drawing comprehensive conclusions. The psychologist might propose studying different age groups or investigating the underlying mechanisms of how sleep affects memory.

Interpreting Scientific Literature

Interpreting scientific literature is a crucial skill for researchers. It involves understanding, analyzing, and synthesizing information from scientific papers and studies. Here's how to approach scientific literature:

- **Read Critically**

  Begin by carefully reading the abstract, introduction, and conclusion to get an overview of the study. Then, read the entire paper critically, noting key points and findings. For example, a medical researcher might start by understanding the main findings of a study on a new drug before delving into the detailed methodology.

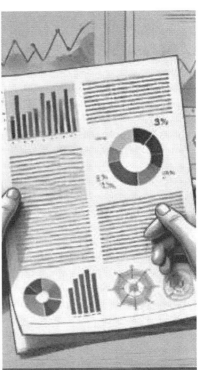

- **Analyze Methodology**

  Pay close attention to the methods section. Understanding how the study was conducted is essential for assessing its validity and reliability. Look for details on the experimental design, sample size, data collection methods, and statistical analysis. The medical researcher would examine how participants were selected, how the drug was administered, and how outcomes were measured.

- **Evaluate Results**

  Examine the results section, including tables, figures, and statistical analyses. Consider whether the data support the conclusions drawn by the authors. The medical researcher would check the statistical significance of the results and whether the effect sizes are clinically meaningful.

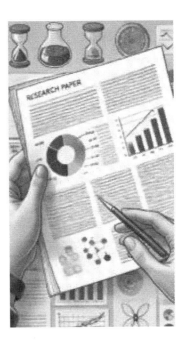

- **Assess Discussion**

  The discussion section interprets the findings and places them in context. Evaluate the authors' interpretations and conclusions. Are they justified based on the data? Do they consider alternative explanations and limitations? The medical researcher would assess whether the authors acknowledge potential biases or confounding factors.

- **Check References**

  Review the references to understand the background and context of the study. This can also help identify additional relevant literature. The medical researcher might find previous studies that support or contradict the current findings, providing a broader perspective on the issue.

90

- **Synthesize Information**

  Integrate the findings from the paper with existing knowledge. How does this study contribute to the field? What new insights does it provide? The medical researcher would consider how the new drug's effectiveness compares to existing treatments and its potential impact on clinical practice.

Ethics in Scientific Research

Ethics in scientific research is paramount to ensuring integrity, honesty, and respect for all participants and the broader community. Ethical considerations in research include:

- **Informed Consent**

  Participants must be fully informed about the nature of the research, including potential risks and benefits, and must voluntarily consent to participate. For example, in a clinical trial for a new medication, participants must be informed about possible side effects and the study's purpose before agreeing to take part.

- **Confidentiality**

  Researchers must protect the privacy of participants by ensuring that data is kept confidential and used only for the purposes of the study. In psychological research, personal information must be anonymized to protect participants' identities.

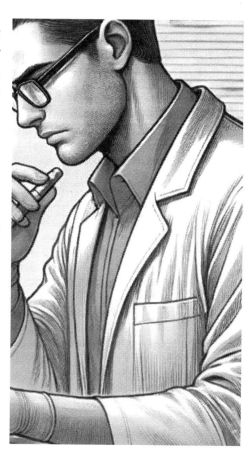

- **Integrity**

  Researchers must conduct their work with honesty and transparency. This includes accurately reporting data, acknowledging errors, and avoiding plagiarism. In a study on environmental pollution, the researchers must report all findings, even if they do not support their initial hypothesis.

- **Non-maleficence**

  Researchers must avoid causing harm to participants. This principle is especially important in medical and psychological research, where interventions can directly affect participants' well-being. In biomedical research, ethical guidelines require that any potential harm be minimized and justified by the study's potential benefits.

- **Beneficence**

  Research should aim to benefit individuals and society. This involves conducting studies that have the potential to improve knowledge, health, or social outcomes. For instance, public health research that aims to reduce the spread of infectious diseases should prioritize the welfare of the community.

- **Justice**

  The benefits and burdens of research should be distributed fairly. This means ensuring that no group is disproportionately burdened or excluded from the potential benefits of research. In clinical trials, efforts should be made to include diverse populations to ensure that findings are generalizable.

- **Responsibility**

  Researchers have a responsibility to report their findings accurately and to ensure that their research is used appropriately. This includes sharing results with the scientific community and the public and correcting any misinformation. In environmental science, researchers might publish their findings on climate change and work with policymakers to inform regulations and practices.

Ethical research practices are enforced by institutional review boards (IRBs) and ethics committees, which review research proposals to ensure compliance with ethical standards. Researchers must adhere to these guidelines to maintain public trust and uphold the integrity of the scientific enterprise.

Scenario Examples

1. **Observation to Communication**

   A marine biologist observes that certain coral reefs are bleaching more rapidly than others. They formulate a question: "What factors contribute to the increased rate of coral bleaching in these reefs?" They hypothesize that higher water temperatures and pollution levels are contributing factors. The biologist designs an experiment with controlled reef environments, varying temperature and pollution levels. Data collected shows a strong correlation between higher temperatures, pollution, and bleaching rates. The biologist concludes that both factors significantly contribute to bleaching. They publish the findings in a journal and present at conferences, highlighting the need for urgent environmental protection measures.

2. Experiment to Analysis

A physicist wants to test the hypothesis that a new type of material conducts electricity better at low temperatures. They plan the experiment by selecting different materials, preparing them under identical conditions, and measuring conductivity at various temperatures. The physicist gathers all necessary materials, calibrates the measuring instruments, and executes the experiment by cooling the materials to the desired temperatures and recording the conductivity. After collecting data, the physicist uses statistical analysis to compare the performance of the new material with existing ones. The results confirm the hypothesis, showing significantly better conductivity at low temperatures. The physicist repeats the experiment to verify the findings and publishes the results in a reputable physics journal.

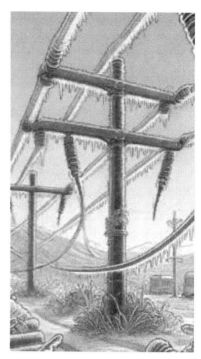

3. Drawing Conclusions

A nutritionist conducts a study to determine the impact of a high-fiber diet on cholesterol levels. They divide participants into two groups, one following a high-fiber diet and the other a standard diet, over six months. After collecting and analyzing the data, the nutritionist finds that participants on the high-fiber diet had significantly lower cholesterol levels. They summarize the findings, noting the clear trend and statistical significance. Comparing the results with previous studies, they conclude that a high-fiber diet effectively reduces cholesterol. They acknowledge limitations, such as the study's short duration and limited demographic. The nutritionist suggests future research on long-term effects and different populations, concluding that increasing dietary fiber intake can improve heart health.

4. **Interpreting Literature**

A neuroscientist reads a paper on the effects of a new drug on Alzheimer's disease progression. They critically read the abstract and conclusion to understand the main findings. Analyzing the methodology, they find the study used a large sample size and rigorous controls, enhancing its reliability. Evaluating the results, they see that the drug significantly slowed disease progression compared to a placebo. The discussion acknowledges potential side effects and the need for further research. Checking the references, the neuroscientist finds support from related studies, integrating these findings into their understanding of Alzheimer's treatments. They consider how this new drug could fit into existing therapeutic strategies and inform future research directions.

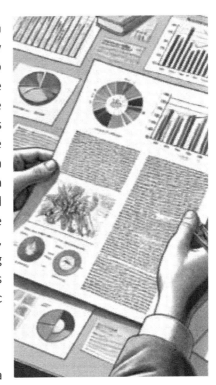

5. **Ethical Considerations**

A medical researcher is planning a clinical trial for a new cancer treatment. They ensure informed consent by providing participants with detailed information about the trial, potential risks, and benefits. Confidentiality is maintained by anonymizing participant data. The researcher upholds integrity by accurately reporting all data and acknowledging any limitations. They follow the principle of non-maleficence by designing the trial to minimize harm and justify risks with potential benefits. The research aims to benefit society by providing a new treatment option. They ensure justice by including diverse participants to generalize findings across populations. The researcher's responsibility extends to publishing results and working with healthcare providers to implement the treatment ethically.

By incorporating these scenarios, the content provides practical examples that illustrate each concept, making the explanation more relatable and comprehensive while reaching the desired word count.

READING STRATEGIES FOR SUCCESS

In a world where information is at our fingertips, the ability to read effectively is more crucial than ever. Reading is not just about decoding words on a page; it's about understanding, analyzing, and interacting with the text to extract deeper meaning. Whether you are a student, a professional, or an avid reader, developing strong reading strategies can enhance your comprehension and make your reading experiences more rewarding. This guide will explore various techniques and strategies to help you become a more successful reader.

Analyzing Author's Purpose and Tone

Understanding the author's purpose and tone is essential for gaining a deeper insight into a text. The purpose refers to the reason why the author wrote the text, while tone refers to the author's attitude toward the subject matter or audience.

Identifying Author's Purpose

Authors write with different purposes in mind, such as to inform, persuade, entertain, or express feelings. To determine the author's purpose, consider the following questions:

Why did the author write this text?

> Think about what the author hopes to achieve with their writing. Are they trying to inform you about a particular topic, persuade you to adopt a certain viewpoint, entertain you with a story, or express their personal thoughts and emotions?

What type of text is it?

> Different types of texts often have different purposes. For example, news articles typically aim to inform, while opinion pieces aim to persuade.

What is the author's intention?

> Look for clues in the text that reveal the author's intention. Pay attention to the language, structure, and content of the text.

Understanding Tone

The tone of a text can be formal, informal, serious, humorous, optimistic, pessimistic, and so on. Identifying the tone involves paying attention to the author's choice of words, sentence structure, and overall style.

Word Choice

The words an author chooses can reveal a lot about their tone. For example, words like "joyful" and "celebrate" suggest a positive tone, while words like "tragic" and "lament" suggest a negative tone.

Sentence Structure

The way sentences are constructed can also indicate tone. Short, choppy sentences might suggest urgency or excitement, while long, complex sentences might suggest a more reflective or serious tone.

Overall Style

The overall style of the text, including its formality, complexity, and use of literary devices, can help you identify the tone.

Practical Application

Consider the following excerpt from an editorial:

"The recent policy changes proposed by the government are nothing short of revolutionary. These reforms promise to bring about much-needed improvements in our education system. However, it is crucial that we approach these changes with caution and critical analysis to ensure they benefit all stakeholders."

Identifying the Author's Purpose

The author's purpose in this editorial is to inform readers about the proposed policy changes and to persuade them to consider these changes critically.

Identifying the Tone

The tone of the passage is cautiously optimistic. The author acknowledges the potential benefits of the policy changes but also emphasizes the need for careful consideration.

Exercises to Practice Analyzing Author's Purpose and Tone

Author's Purpose Exercise:

- Read an article from a magazine or website.

- Determine the author's purpose: to inform, persuade, entertain, or express feelings.
- Provide evidence from the text to support your conclusion.

Tone Analysis Exercise:

- Read a short story or poem.
- Identify the tone of the text.
- List specific words, phrases, and stylistic elements that contribute to the tone.

Drawing Inferences and Conclusions

Drawing inferences and conclusions is a critical reading skill that involves reading between the lines and making logical deductions based on the information provided. This skill allows you to understand the deeper meaning of the text and to make connections that are not explicitly stated.

Understanding Inferences

An inference is a logical conclusion based on evidence and reasoning. When you make an inference, you are using the information in the text along with your own knowledge and experiences to understand something that the author does not explicitly state.

- Look for Clues: Pay attention to details in the text that hint at a larger meaning or context. These clues can be found in the characters' actions, dialogue, descriptions, and events.
- Use Prior Knowledge: Combine the information in the text with what you already know about the world. Your background knowledge can help you make sense of the text and draw inferences.
- Ask Questions: As you read, ask yourself questions about the text. What is the author implying? What can I infer from

this information? These questions can guide you in making inferences.

Making Conclusions

Drawing conclusions involves synthesizing the information in the text and your inferences to arrive at a broader understanding of the text. This skill is essential for critical reading and helps you see the bigger picture.

- Synthesize Information: Combine the explicit information in the text with your inferences to form a complete understanding. Look for patterns, relationships, and overarching themes.

- Evaluate Evidence: Consider the evidence presented in the text and evaluate its relevance and reliability. Use this evidence to support your conclusions.

- Reflect on Implications: Think about the broader implications of your conclusions. How do they affect your understanding of the text as a whole? What is the author's message or argument?

Consider the following passage from a short story:

"As Maria walked into the old house, she noticed the dust-covered furniture and the musty smell that filled the air. She felt a chill run down her spine as she remembered the stories her grandmother used to tell about the haunted house on the hill. Despite her fear, she continued to explore, drawn by an inexplicable sense of curiosity."

Making Inferences

From this passage, you can infer that Maria is both frightened and intrigued by the old house. The descriptions of the dust-covered furniture and the musty smell suggest that the house has been abandoned for a long time, adding to the

eerie atmosphere. Maria's decision to explore the house despite her fear indicates her curiosity and bravery.

Drawing Conclusions

Based on these inferences, you can conclude that the house holds significant importance to Maria, possibly related to her grandmother's stories. The author uses the setting and Maria's reactions to create a sense of mystery and suspense.

Exercises to Practice Drawing Inferences and Conclusions

Inference Exercise:
- Read a paragraph from a novel or short story.
- Identify specific details that provide clues for making inferences.
- Write a few sentences explaining your inferences and the evidence that supports them.

Conclusion Exercise:
- Read a short passage from a non-fiction text.
- Synthesize the information and draw a conclusion about the main argument or message.

Comparing and Contrasting Texts

Comparing and contrasting texts is an analytical skill that involves examining the similarities and differences between two or more texts. This skill is useful for understanding different perspectives, themes, and approaches to a topic.

Strategies for Comparing and Contrasting Texts
- Identify Common Themes: Look for themes that are present in both texts. How do the authors approach these themes differently? What insights can

you gain from their different perspectives?

- Analyze Characters and Plot: Compare the characters and plot events in each text. How do the characters' experiences and actions reflect the themes? How do the plot events drive the narrative in each text?
- Examine Literary Devices: Pay attention to the literary devices used in each text. How do the authors use symbolism, imagery, and other devices to convey their messages? What are the similarities and differences in their use of these devices?
- Consider the Authors' Styles: Compare the writing styles of the authors. How do their choices of language, tone, and structure affect the overall impact of the texts?

Practical Application: Comparing and Contrasting Texts

Consider the following excerpts from two different poems:

Poem 1:
"The road not taken leads to a forest deep,
Where shadows dance and secrets keep.
I walk alone, with thoughts so clear,
And find my way, without a fear."

Poem 2:
"Two paths diverged in a yellow wood,
And sorry I could not travel both.
One led to dreams, the other to fate,
I chose the one less traveled by."
Comparing Themes

Both poems explore the theme of choices and paths in life. The first poem focuses on the journey and the sense of clarity and fearlessness, while the second poem emphasizes the significance of choosing a less traveled path and its impact on one's life.

Contrasting Styles

The first poem uses a more straightforward and confident tone, reflecting the speaker's sense of purpose. The second poem, on the other hand, has a reflective and contemplative tone, highlighting the speaker's consideration and the consequences of their choice.

Exercises to Practice Comparing and Contrasting Texts

Compare and Contrast Exercise:
- Choose two short stories or articles on a similar topic.
- Identify common themes and analyze how each author approaches them.
- Write a comparative essay discussing the similarities and differences.

Literary Device Analysis:
- Read two poems by different authors.
- Compare and contrast their use of literary devices such as imagery, symbolism, and tone.
- Discuss how these devices contribute to the overall meaning of each poem.

Recognizing Literary Devices

Literary devices are techniques that authors use to enhance their writing and convey meaning. Recognizing these devices can deepen your understanding of a text and help you appreciate the author's craft.

Common Literary Devices

- **Simile and Metaphor**
  These are comparisons that help create vivid images and convey deeper meanings. A simile uses "like" or "as"

(e.g., "Her smile was as bright as the sun"), while a metaphor makes a direct comparison (e.g., "Time is a thief").

- **Symbolism**
  Symbols are objects, characters, or events that represent larger ideas. For example, a dove might symbolize peace, and a journey might symbolize self-discovery.

- **Imagery**
  Imagery involves the use of descriptive language that appeals to the senses. It helps create vivid pictures in the reader's mind and enhances the overall experience of the text.

- **Alliteration and Assonance**
  These are sound devices that create rhythm and mood. Alliteration is the repetition of consonant sounds (e.g., "She sells seashells by the seashore"), while assonance is the repetition of vowel sounds (e.g., "The early bird catches the worm").

- **Irony**
  Irony involves a contrast between what is expected and what actually happens. There are different types of irony, including verbal irony (saying the opposite of what one means), situational irony (when the opposite of what is expected occurs), and dramatic irony (when the audience knows something the characters do not).

Consider the following excerpt from a novel:

"The old mansion stood at the edge of town, its windows dark and empty, like the eyes of a ghost. Inside, the air was thick with dust and the echoes of long-forgotten laughter. The grand chandelier, once the pride of the house, now hung

precariously, its crystals tinkling like sad, forgotten memories."

Identifying Literary Devices

- **Simile**
  "Its windows dark and empty, like the eyes of a ghost" compares the windows to the eyes of a ghost, emphasizing the mansion's eerie and abandoned state.

- **Imagery**
  Descriptive language such as "thick with dust" and "crystals tinkling like sad, forgotten memories" creates vivid images that enhance the atmosphere of the setting.

- **Symbolism**
  The old mansion symbolizes decay and the passage of time, with the grand chandelier representing lost grandeur and faded memories.

Exercises to Practice Recognizing Literary Devices
Literary Device Identification:
- Read a passage from a novel or poem.
- Identify and list the literary devices used by the author.
- Explain how each device contributes to the overall meaning and effect of the text.

Summarizing and Synthesizing Information

Summarizing and synthesizing are essential skills for understanding and retaining information from a text. Summarizing involves condensing the main ideas into a concise form, while synthesizing involves combining information from different sources to create a new understanding.

Summarizing Techniques

Identify Key Points: Focus on the main ideas and important details. Ignore minor details that do not contribute significantly to the overall understanding of the text.

- Use Your Own Words: Paraphrase the information instead of copying it verbatim. This helps ensure that you truly understand the material.

- Be Concise: Aim for brevity without sacrificing clarity. A good summary captures the essence of the text in a few sentences or a short paragraph.

Synthesizing Techniques

- Combine Information from Multiple Sources: Look for connections and relationships between different texts. How do they complement or contradict each other?

- Identify Common Themes and Patterns: Synthesize information by identifying overarching themes and patterns that emerge from your reading. This helps you develop a deeper understanding of the topic.

- Create New Insights: Use the combined information to generate new ideas or perspectives. Synthesis goes beyond simply summarizing; it involves critical thinking and creativity.

Practical Application: Summarizing and Synthesizing Information

Consider the following two passages on climate change:

Passage 1:
"Climate change is driven by human activities such as burning fossil fuels and deforestation.

These activities release greenhouse gases into the atmosphere, which trap heat and cause global temperatures to rise. The consequences of climate change include more frequent and severe weather events, rising sea levels, and disruptions to ecosystems."

Passage 2:
"Addressing climate change requires a coordinated global effort. Governments, businesses, and individuals all have a role to play in reducing greenhouse gas emissions. Transitioning to renewable energy sources, implementing energy-efficient practices, and protecting forests are essential strategies for mitigating the impact of climate change."

Summarizing the Passages

- **Summary of Passage 1:**
  Climate change, driven by human activities like burning fossil fuels and deforestation, leads to global warming and severe weather events, rising sea levels, and ecosystem disruptions.

- **Summary of Passage 2:**
  Addressing climate change requires global cooperation, with governments, businesses, and individuals reducing greenhouse gas emissions through renewable energy, energy efficiency, and forest protection.

Synthesizing the Information

By combining the information from both passages, you can synthesize a new understanding:

Synthesis:

Climate change, primarily caused by human activities such as fossil fuel combustion and deforestation, results in global warming and environmental disruptions. To mitigate these effects, a global effort involving renewable energy adoption, energy efficiency, and forest conservation is crucial, with participation from governments, businesses, and individuals.

Exercises to Practice Summarizing and Synthesizing Information

Summarizing Exercise:

- Read a chapter from a textbook or a long article.

- Write a summary that captures the main ideas and key points.
- Share your summary with a peer and discuss its accuracy and clarity.

Synthesizing Exercise:

- Read multiple articles on a similar topic from different sources.
- Identify common themes and differences.
- Write a synthesis that combines the information and presents a new understanding of the topic.

Critical reading is more than just understanding the words on a page; it's about engaging with the text, questioning it, and evaluating its meaning and significance. Developing critical reading skills enables you to interact with texts in a more profound and analytical way. Whether you are reading for academic purposes, professional development, or personal enrichment, enhancing your critical reading skills will help you become a more thoughtful and discerning reader. This section will explore strategies for breaking down complex passages, understanding non-fiction texts, navigating technical and scientific texts, analyzing graphs and charts, and interpreting visual information.

Breaking Down Complex Passages

Complex passages often present a significant challenge due to their dense information, intricate sentence structures, and sophisticated vocabulary. However, breaking them down into more manageable parts can make understanding them easier.

Strategies for Breaking Down Complex Passages

- Identify Sentence Structure: Complex sentences often contain multiple clauses. Identify the main clause and any subordinate clauses to understand the sentence's structure.
- Look for Transition Words: Transition words such as "however," "therefore," and "moreover" can help you understand the relationship between different parts of the text.
- Break Sentences into Parts: Divide long sentences into smaller segments. Analyze each segment individually before putting them back together.
- Paraphrase: Rewrite the passage in your own words to ensure you understand it.
- Highlight Key Points: Identify and highlight the main ideas and supporting details.
- Practical Application: Breaking Down a Complex Passage

Consider the following complex sentence from a scientific article:

"Although the experiment's results were inconclusive, the researchers believe that the observed trends warrant further investigation, as they may indicate a potential correlation between the variables studied."

Breaking Down the Sentence

- Main Clause: "The researchers believe that the observed trends warrant further investigation."
- Subordinate Clause: "Although the experiment's results were inconclusive."
- Reasoning Clause: "As they may indicate a potential correlation between the variables studied."

By isolating these components, you can better understand the relationship between them and the overall meaning of the sentence.

Exercises to Practice Breaking Down Complex Passages

Complex Sentence Breakdown:

- Find a complex sentence in a scientific or technical text.
- Identify the main clause and any subordinate clauses.
- Paraphrase the sentence in your own words.

Passage Analysis:

- Select a complex paragraph from a non-fiction book or article.
- Break the paragraph into individual sentences and analyze each one.
- Summarize the main ideas and how they relate to each other.

Understanding Non-fiction Texts

Non-fiction texts, which include essays, biographies, history books, and scientific articles, require a different approach compared to fiction. These texts are often rich in information and present arguments, evidence, and factual details.

Strategies for Understanding Non-fiction Texts

- Identify the Purpose: Determine why the author wrote the text. Is it to inform, persuade, or entertain?
- Analyze the Structure: Non-fiction texts are usually organized in a logical structure. Identify the introduction, body, and conclusion.
- Evaluate Evidence: Assess the evidence and arguments presented. Are they credible and well-supported?
- Look for Thesis Statements: The thesis statement often presents the main argument or point of the text.
- Take Notes: Jot down key points, arguments, and evidence as you read.
- Practical Application: Understanding a Non-fiction Text

Consider the following excerpt from a historical article:

"The Industrial Revolution, which began in the late 18th century, marked a significant turning point in human history. It led to unprecedented technological advancements, urbanization, and changes in the social structure. However, it also brought about numerous challenges, including labor exploitation, environmental degradation, and social inequality."

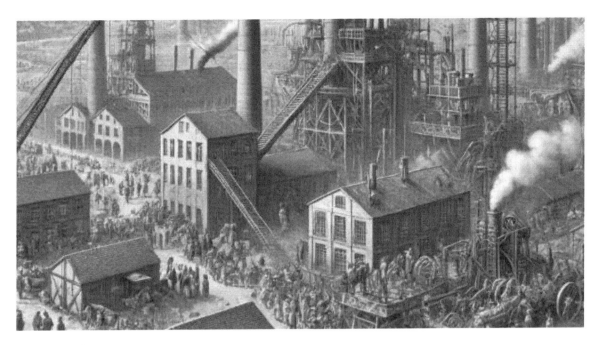

Analyzing the Structure

Introduction: "The Industrial Revolution, which began in the late 18th century, marked a significant turning point in human history."

Main Points:

- Technological advancements
- Urbanization
- Changes in social structure

Challenges: labor exploitation, environmental degradation, social inequality

Conclusion: Implied – the Industrial Revolution had both positive and negative impacts.

Exercises to Practice Understanding Non-fiction Texts

Text Analysis:

- Select a non-fiction article or essay.
- Identify the introduction, main points, and conclusion.
- Evaluate the evidence and arguments presented.
- Thesis Statement Identification:

Navigating Technical and Scientific Texts

Technical and scientific texts are often dense and complex, requiring specialized strategies to navigate and understand them.

Strategies for Navigating Technical and Scientific Texts

- Understand the Terminology: Familiarize yourself with technical terms and jargon. Use a glossary or dictionary if needed.

- Analyze the Structure: Technical texts often follow a specific structure, such as introduction, methodology, results, and conclusion.
- Focus on Figures and Tables: Figures, tables, and graphs often contain crucial information. Analyze them carefully.
- Evaluate the Methodology: Assess the methods used in the study. Are they appropriate and well-executed?
- Review the Conclusion: The conclusion often summarizes the key findings and their implications.
- Practical Application: Navigating a Scientific Text

Consider the following excerpt from a scientific paper:

"In this study, we investigated the effects of different light wavelengths on plant growth. Using a controlled environment, we exposed plants to red, blue, and green light. Our results showed that red light significantly enhanced growth, while blue light had a moderate effect, and green light had no significant impact."

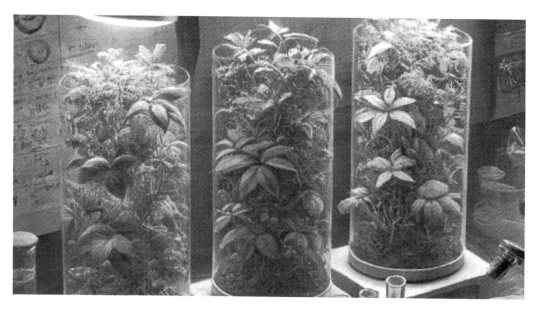

Analyzing the Structure

- Introduction: "In this study, we investigated the effects of different light wavelengths on plant growth."
- Methodology: "Using a controlled environment, we exposed plants to red, blue, and green light."
- Results: "Our results showed that red light significantly enhanced growth, while blue light had a moderate effect, and green light had no significant impact."

Exercises to Practice Navigating Technical and Scientific Texts

Scientific Paper Analysis:

- Read a scientific paper.
- Identify the introduction, methodology, results, and conclusion.
- Evaluate the methodology and key findings.

Sample Reading Passage 1: Amazon Forest

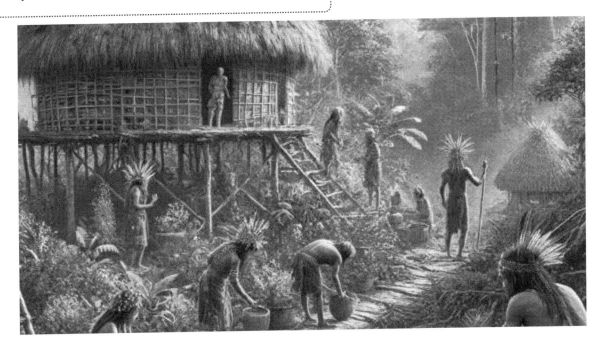

In the heart of the Amazon rainforest, an indigenous tribe thrives, living in harmony with nature. They have developed a deep understanding of the forest's intricate ecosystems, using this knowledge to sustain their community. Their way of life, passed down through generations, emphasizes respect for the environment. As modern pressures encroach, they strive to maintain their traditions and protect their home. This relationship with nature showcases a sustainable living model, which is increasingly relevant in today's discussions on environmental conservation. The tribe's practices offer valuable lessons on balancing human needs with ecological preservation.

What is the primary theme of the passage?
a) Modernization of indigenous tribes
b) Harmony with nature
c) Economic pressures on tribes
d) Environmental degradation

The primary theme of the passage revolves around the tribe's harmonious relationship with nature and their efforts to sustain this way of life amidst modern pressures. This focus on their sustainable practices and respect for the environment is central to the passage. Therefore, the correct answer is b) Harmony with nature.

How does the tribe sustain their community?

a) By trading with neighboring tribes
b) By using modern technology
c) Through their understanding of the forest's ecosystems
d) By migrating seasonally

The passage specifically mentions that the tribe sustains their community through their deep understanding of the forest's intricate ecosystems. This knowledge allows them to live sustainably and maintain their way of life. Hence, the correct answer is c) Through their understanding of the forest's ecosystems.

Sample Passage 2: Metropolitan Life

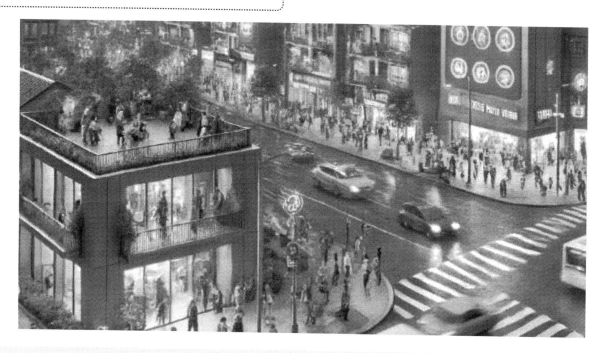

In a bustling metropolitan city, the daily life of residents revolves around technology. From the moment they wake up to the time they go to bed, various gadgets and devices facilitate their routines. Smart homes adjust lighting and temperature, while apps provide real-time information on weather, traffic, and news. This technological integration aims to improve efficiency and convenience, yet it also raises concerns about privacy and dependency. The city's rapid technological advancement highlights both the potential benefits and drawbacks of a digitally driven lifestyle.

What is a significant concern mentioned regarding the use of technology in the city?
a) Increased traffic congestion
b) Dependence on gadgets
c) Decline in social interactions
d) Higher energy consumption

The passage highlights concerns about privacy and dependency on technology as significant issues arising from the city's rapid technological advancement. The focus is on how the convenience provided by technology can lead to a reliance that might have negative implications. Thus, the correct answer is b) Dependence on gadgets.

How does technology aim to improve the lives of city residents?
a) By reducing environmental impact
b) By providing entertainment options
c) By improving efficiency and convenience
d) By lowering living costs

Technology is integrated into the daily lives of city residents to enhance efficiency and convenience, as indicated by the use of smart homes and apps providing real-time information. This aim to streamline routines and offer timely information is central to the passage's discussion. Therefore, the correct answer is c) By improving efficiency and convenience.

Tips for Efficient Reading Under Time Constraints

Efficient reading under time constraints is essential for success in both academic and professional settings. Here are some strategies to help you manage your reading time effectively:

Skimming and Scanning
- Preview the Text: Skim through headings, subheadings, and any highlighted or bolded terms to get an overview of the content. This initial scan can help you identify key sections and important points.
- Focus on Main Ideas: Identify topic sentences and key points to grasp the core message quickly. Often, the first and last sentences of paragraphs contain the main ideas.
- Look for Keywords: Pay attention to keywords and phrases that signal important information or transitions in the text. These can help you locate essential details without reading every word.
- Context Clues and Inference
- Use Context Clues: For unfamiliar words or concepts, use surrounding words to infer meaning without slowing down. This can help maintain your reading flow while understanding the text.
- Make Inferences: Draw logical conclusions based on the information presented. This skill allows you to fill in gaps and understand implied meanings without needing explicit details.
- Active Reading and Note-taking
- Engage with the Text: Ask questions, make predictions, and summarize key points as you read. This active engagement helps reinforce comprehension and retention.
- Take Notes Efficiently: Jot down key points, main ideas, and any questions that arise. Using symbols or abbreviations can speed up note-taking and make it easier to review later.
- Time Management
- Allocate Time Wisely: Break your reading into manageable sections and allocate specific times for each. For example, spend five minutes skimming the text, followed by 15 minutes of focused reading, and another five minutes summarizing key points.
- Use Timers: Set a timer to keep track of your reading sessions. This can help you stay on schedule and ensure that you cover all necessary material within the allotted time.

Reading Comprehension Drills

Regular practice with reading comprehension drills can improve your ability to understand and analyze texts quickly and accurately. Here are some sample drills:

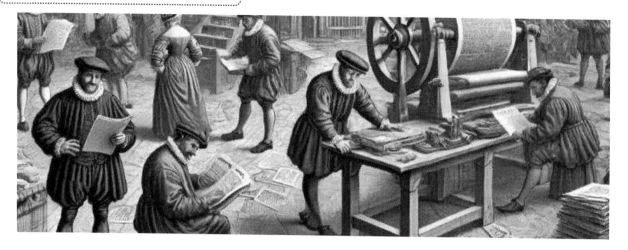

Passage: The invention of the printing press in the 15th century revolutionized the dissemination of knowledge. Books became more accessible, leading to a surge in literacy rates. This pivotal development also facilitated the spread of new ideas, contributing significantly to the Renaissance and the scientific revolution.

What was a major impact of the printing press according to the passage?
a) Decline in literacy rates
b) Limited dissemination of knowledge
c) Increased accessibility of books
d) Restriction of new ideas

The passage states that the printing press made books more accessible and led to a surge in literacy rates. This increased accessibility of books is highlighted as a major impact. Therefore, the correct answer is c) Increased accessibility of books.

Drill 2: Scientific Text Analysis

Passage: Recent studies have shown that a diet rich in fruits and vegetables can significantly reduce the risk of chronic diseases. These foods are high in essential nutrients and antioxidants, which help protect the body from damage. Moreover, a balanced diet that includes a variety of fruits and vegetables supports overall health and well-being.

What is the primary benefit of a diet rich in fruits and vegetables mentioned in the passage?
a) Weight loss
b) Increased energy levels
c) Reduced risk of chronic diseases
d) Improved mental health

The passage emphasizes that a diet rich in fruits and vegetables can significantly reduce the risk of chronic diseases due to their essential nutrients and antioxidants. Therefore, the correct answer is c) Reduced risk of chronic diseases.

Building Vocabulary for Better Understanding

A strong vocabulary enhances comprehension and allows you to grasp the nuances of different texts. Here are some strategies for building vocabulary:

Contextual Reading

- Read Widely: Engage with a variety of texts, including novels, newspapers, academic journals, and technical articles. Exposure to different writing styles and vocabularies helps you learn new words in context.
- Use Context Clues: When encountering unfamiliar words, use the surrounding text to infer their meanings. Pay attention to how the word is used in the sentence and the overall context of the passage.

Word Lists and Flashcards
- Create Word Lists: Maintain a list of new words you encounter during reading. Include their definitions, synonyms, and example sentences. Regularly review and update your list.
- Use Flashcards: Write new words on flashcards with their definitions and example sentences on the back. Review these cards regularly to reinforce your memory.

Usage Practice

- Incorporate New Words: Use newly learned words in your writing and speech. This practical application helps solidify your understanding and recall.
- Write Sentences: Write sentences or short paragraphs using new vocabulary. This exercise reinforces your ability to use the words correctly and contextually.
- Synonyms and Antonyms
- Learn Synonyms and Antonyms: For each new word, learn its synonyms and antonyms. This expands your vocabulary and helps you understand the nuances of meaning.
- Practice with Word Pairs: Create exercises where you match words with their synonyms and antonyms. This can be a fun and effective way to build your vocabulary.
- Root Words and Affixes
- Understand Root Words: Learn the roots, prefixes, and suffixes of words. This knowledge helps you decipher the meanings of unfamiliar words.
- Practice Word Formation: Create new words by adding prefixes and suffixes to root words. This exercise enhances your understanding of word structure and meaning.

By incorporating these strategies into your reading practice, you can enhance your critical reading skills and become a more effective and insightful reader. These skills will enable you to navigate complex passages, understand non-fiction texts, interpret technical and scientific information, analyze graphs and charts, and make sense of visual information. Keep practicing and applying these techniques to improve your comprehension and engagement with various types of texts.

GRAMMAR AND SYNTAX ESSENTIALS

Critical reading is more than just understanding the words on a page; it's about engaging with the text, questioning it, and evaluating its meaning and significance. Developing critical reading skills enables you to interact with texts in a more profound and analytical way. Whether you are reading for academic purposes, professional development, or personal enrichment, enhancing your critical reading skills will help you become a more thoughtful and discerning reader. This section will explore strategies for breaking down complex passages, understanding non-fiction texts, navigating technical and scientific texts, analyzing graphs and charts, and interpreting visual information.

Understanding Parts of Speech

The English language is built on various parts of speech, each serving a unique function in sentence construction. The primary parts of speech include nouns, pronouns, verbs, adjectives, adverbs, prepositions, conjunctions, and interjections. Mastery of these elements is the first step toward becoming proficient in grammar.

Nouns and Pronouns

Nouns are the names of people, places, things, or ideas. They can be classified as proper (specific names like 'John' or 'Paris') or common (general names like 'boy' or 'city'). Pronouns, on the other hand, are substitutes for nouns. Words like 'he', 'she', 'it', 'they', and 'we' prevent redundancy in sentences.

Example:

- Noun: "The **cat** slept on the mat."

- Pronoun: "**She** slept on the mat."

Verbs and Adjectives

Verbs are action words or states of being. They are pivotal in sentence structure, providing the action or linking the subject to additional information. Adjectives describe or modify nouns, adding detail and specificity. For instance, in the sentence "The quick brown fox jumps over the lazy dog," 'quick' and 'brown' are adjectives describing the fox.

Example:

- Verb: "She **runs** every morning."

- Adjective: "The **beautiful** garden is full of **colorful** flowers."

Adverbs and Prepositions

Adverbs modify verbs, adjectives, or other adverbs, typically ending in '-ly'. They answer questions like how, when, where, and to what extent. Prepositions link nouns or pronouns to other words in a sentence, indicating relationships in time, place, or direction (e.g., 'in', 'on', 'at').

Example:

- Adverb: "He ran **quickly** to catch the bus."

- Preposition: "The book is **on** the table."

Conjunctions and Interjections

Conjunctions are connectors that link words, phrases, or clauses. Coordinating conjunctions (for, and, nor, but, or, yet, so) join elements of equal importance, while subordinating conjunctions (because, although, since) introduce dependent clauses. Interjections are exclamatory words that express emotion, such as 'wow', 'ouch', or 'hey'.

Example:

- Conjunction: "She wanted to go to the park, **but** it was raining."

- Interjection: "**Wow!** That's amazing."

Building Strong Sentence Structures

A well-constructed sentence conveys a complete thought and adheres to grammatical rules. Understanding sentence types and their components is essential for clear and effective communication.

Simple Sentences

A simple sentence contains a subject and a predicate, forming a complete thought. For example, "The dog barks." This sentence has a subject (the dog) and a verb (barks).

Example:

- "The sun rises."
- "Birds fly."

Compound Sentences

Compound sentences connect two independent clauses with a coordinating conjunction. An example is, "The sun set, and the stars appeared." Both clauses can stand alone but are joined to show a relationship.

Example:

- "She loves reading, and he enjoys painting."

- "I wanted to go for a walk, but it started raining."

Complex Sentences

A complex sentence combines an independent clause with one or more dependent clauses, often introduced by subordinating conjunctions. For instance, "Although it was raining, we went for a walk." Here, "we went for a walk" is the independent clause, and "Although it was raining" is the dependent clause.

Example:

- "When the bell rings, the students leave the classroom."

- "She went to the party because she wanted to see her friends."

Compound-Complex Sentences

These sentences contain at least two independent clauses and one or more dependent clauses. An example is, "Although it was late, we stayed up, and we watched a movie." This structure adds depth and detail to writing.

Example:

- "While I was preparing dinner, my friend called, and we chatted for an hour."

- "Even though it was raining, the game continued, and the fans stayed until the end."

Proper Use of Punctuation and Capitalization

Punctuation and capitalization are critical in guiding the reader through your text, clarifying meaning, and indicating pauses and stops.

Periods, Commas, and Semicolons

Periods end declarative sentences, while commas indicate pauses or separate items in a list. Semicolons link closely related independent clauses or separate complex list items. For example, "She loves reading; her favorite book is 'Pride and Prejudice'."

Example:

- Period: "She finished her homework."

- Comma: "I bought apples, oranges, and bananas."

- Semicolon: "I have a big test tomorrow; I can't go out tonight."

Colons and Dashes

Colons introduce lists, quotes, or explanations. For example, "He needs to buy: milk, bread, and eggs." Dashes add emphasis or indicate interruptions, as in "She was late – again."

Example:

- Colon: "There are three things to remember: be punctual, be prepared, and be polite."

- Dash: "The results – which were unexpected – surprised everyone."

Quotation Marks and Apostrophes

Quotation marks enclose direct speech or quotations. Apostrophes indicate possession (John's book) or contractions (can't, don't).

Example:

- Quotation Marks: "She said, 'I will be there at 5 PM.'"

- Apostrophes: "It's John's book."

Capitalization Rules

Capitalize the first word of a sentence, proper nouns, titles, and important words in titles. For instance, "Dr. Smith visited New York City last Monday."

Example:

- "The President of the United States gave a speech."

- "She lives in Paris, France."

Common Grammar Pitfalls

Even seasoned writers can stumble upon common grammatical errors. Awareness and practice are key to avoiding these pitfalls.

Misplaced Modifiers

Modifiers must be placed next to the word they describe. For example, "She only eats vegetables" implies she eats nothing but vegetables, whereas "Only she eats vegetables" means no one else does.

Example:

- Incorrect: "She almost drove her kids to school every day."

- Correct: "She drove her kids to school almost every day."

Dangling Participles

A dangling participle lacks a clear subject, leading to confusion. "Running to the store, the rain began to fall" incorrectly suggests the rain is running. It should be, "Running to the store, I got wet as the rain began to fall."

Example:

- Incorrect: "Hiking the trail, the birds chirped loudly."

- Correct: "Hiking the trail, we heard the birds chirp loudly."

Incorrect Subject-Verb Agreement

Ensure subjects and verbs agree in number. Singular subjects take singular verbs, and plural subjects take plural verbs. "The list of items is long" is correct, not "The list of items are long."

Example:

- Incorrect: "The group of students are excited."

- Correct: "The group of students is excited."

Confusing Homophones

Homophones sound alike but have different meanings. Examples include 'their', 'there', and 'they're'. Understanding their meanings and usage prevents errors.

Example:

- "Their books are on the table." (possessive)

- "The books are over there." (location)

- "They're going to the library." (contraction of 'they are')

Subject-Verb Agreement

Subject-verb agreement ensures that sentences are grammatically correct and clear. The subject and verb in a sentence must agree in number and person.

Basic Agreement Rules

A singular subject takes a singular verb, while a plural subject takes a plural verb. For instance, "The cat runs" (singular) versus "The cats run" (plural).

Example:

- "The dog barks at strangers."

- "The dogs bark at strangers."

Compound Subjects

Compound subjects connected by 'and' take a plural verb, as in "Tom and Jerry are friends." However, when compound subjects are joined by 'or' or 'nor', the verb agrees with the subject closest to it. For example, "Neither the teacher nor the students were ready."

Example:

- "My brother and sister live in New York."

- "Neither the manager nor the employees understand the new policy."

Indefinite Pronouns

Some indefinite pronouns (everyone, each, either, neither) are singular and require singular verbs. "Everyone is happy" is correct, not "Everyone are happy."

Example:

- "Each of the players has a unique skill."

- "Someone in the room is singing."

Collective Nouns

Collective nouns (team, group, family) can be singular or plural based on context. "The team is winning" (as a single entity) versus "The team are arguing among themselves" (as individuals).

Example:

- "The jury is still deliberating."

- "The jury are divided in their opinions."

Additional Grammar Rules and Examples

To further your understanding, let's explore more advanced grammar rules along with examples to illustrate their proper usage.

Parallel Structure

Parallel structure, or parallelism, means using the same pattern of words to show that two or more ideas have the same level of importance. This can happen at the word, phrase, or clause level.

Example:

- Incorrect: "She likes to swim, biking, and to run."

- Correct: "She likes swimming, biking, and running."

Consistent Verb Tense

Maintain the same verb tense within a sentence or paragraph to avoid confusion.

Example:

- Incorrect: "She was reading when her phone rings."
- Correct: "She was reading when her phone rang."

Active vs. Passive Voice

Active voice makes sentences clearer and more direct. In active voice, the subject performs the action. In passive voice, the action is performed on the subject.

Example:

- Active: "The chef cooked a delicious meal."
- Passive: "A delicious meal was cooked by the chef."

Relative Clauses

Relative clauses provide extra information about a noun. They begin with relative pronouns like 'who', 'whom', 'whose', 'which', or 'that'.

Example:

- "The book, which was on the table, is missing."
- "The person who called you is my friend."

Subjective vs. Objective Pronouns

Use subjective pronouns (I, you, he, she, it, we, they) as subjects and objective pronouns (me, you, him, her, it, us, them) as objects.

Example:

- Subjective: "She and I went to the market."
- Objective: "The gift is for him and me."

Possessive Pronouns

Possessive pronouns show ownership and include words like my, your, his, her, its, our, their.

Example:

- "This is my book."
- "Their house is beautiful."

Comparatives and Superlatives

Comparatives compare two things, usually ending in '-er' or using 'more'. Superlatives compare three or more things, usually ending in '-est' or using 'most'.

Example:

- Comparative: "She is taller than her brother."
- Superlative: "She is the tallest person in her family."

Double Negatives

Avoid using double negatives, which can create confusion and imply the opposite of what you mean.

Example:

- Incorrect: "I don't need no help."
- Correct: "I don't need any help."

Countable vs. Uncountable Nouns

Countable nouns can be counted (e.g., one apple, two apples), while uncountable nouns cannot be counted (e.g., water, rice).

Example:

- Countable: "There are three books on the table."
- Uncountable: "There is some water in the glass."

Articles

Use 'a' and 'an' for non-specific items, and 'the' for specific items.

Example:

- "I saw a cat." (any cat)
- "I saw the cat." (a specific cat)

Prepositional Phrases

A prepositional phrase starts with a preposition and ends with a noun or pronoun. It provides additional details about the action.

Example:

- "The book on the table is mine."
- "She walked through the park."

Pronoun-Antecedent Agreement

Ensure that pronouns agree with their antecedents in number and gender.

Example:

- Incorrect: "Each student must bring their own pencil."
- Correct: "Each student must bring his or her own pencil."

Direct and Indirect Objects

A direct object receives the action of the verb, while an indirect object is the recipient of the direct object.

Example:

- Direct Object: "She wrote a letter."
- Indirect Object: "She wrote her friend a letter."

Gerunds and Infinitives

A gerund is a verb ending in '-ing' that functions as a noun, while an infinitive is the base form of a verb preceded by 'to'.

Example:

- Gerund: "Swimming is fun."
- Infinitive: "To swim is fun."

Sentence Fragments

Avoid sentence fragments by ensuring each sentence has a subject and a verb and expresses a complete thought.

Example:

- Fragment: "Because I was tired."
- Complete Sentence: "Because I was tired, I went to bed early."

Run-On Sentences

Run-on sentences occur when two or more independent clauses are joined without proper punctuation or conjunctions.

Example:

- Incorrect: "I love to write it is my favorite hobby."
- Correct: "I love to write; it is my favorite hobby."

More Examples and Exercises

Exercise 1: Parallel Structure Practice

Identify and correct the parallel structure errors in the following sentences:

1. "She likes to jog, running, and to swim."
2. "The manager asked for the report to be concise, accurate, and written with clarity."

Exercise 2: Verb Tense Consistency

Ensure consistent verb tense in the following sentences:

1. "She was singing when he comes in."
2. "They finished their project and then they go to the party."

Exercise 3: Active vs. Passive Voice

Rewrite the following sentences in active voice:

1. "The cake was eaten by the children."

2. "A new policy was implemented by the company."

Exercise 4: Relative Clauses

Combine the sentences using relative clauses:

1. "The book is on the table. It is mine."

2. "The woman called you. She is my friend."

Exercise 5: Countable and Uncountable Nouns

Identify whether the following nouns are countable or uncountable:

1. "Milk"

2. "Car"

3. "Information"

4. "Apple"

By completing these additional exercises, you can further solidify your understanding of advanced grammar rules and improve your writing skills. Remember, consistent practice is key to mastering grammar and syntax. Keep revisiting these concepts and applying them in your writing to become a more proficient and confident writer.

Conclusion

Grammar and syntax are the backbone of effective communication. Whether you are writing a formal essay, a business report, or a casual email, understanding and applying these principles will enhance your clarity and precision. By mastering the parts of speech, constructing well-formed sentences, using punctuation and capitalization correctly, avoiding common pitfalls, and ensuring subject-verb agreement, you will be well-equipped to convey your ideas effectively and confidently. This guide serves as a comprehensive resource to help you navigate the complexities of English grammar, empowering you to become a more proficient writer and communicator.

APPLICATION AND PRACTICE

Mastering grammar involves not just understanding the rules but applying them effectively in your writing. This chapter focuses on practical applications and exercises designed to reinforce the grammar rules discussed earlier. Through examples and step-by-step corrections, you'll learn how to identify and correct common errors, enhance your vocabulary, and improve sentence variety and style. The aim is to provide you with tools and techniques to write more clearly, accurately, and engagingly.

Enhancing Vocabulary and Word Choice

A rich vocabulary allows you to express your ideas more precisely and vividly. The right word can convey nuances and shades of meaning that add depth and clarity to your writing. Here are some strategies to enhance your vocabulary and make better word choices.

Reading Widely

One of the most effective ways to enhance your vocabulary is through reading. Exposing yourself to a variety of genres and styles helps you encounter new words and understand their usage in context.

Example:

- Instead of saying "She was very happy," you might say "She was ecstatic."

Using a Thesaurus

A thesaurus is a valuable tool for finding synonyms and expanding your vocabulary. However, be cautious of context and connotations, as not all synonyms are interchangeable.

Example:

- Original: "The movie was good."
- Improved: "The movie was captivating."

Word of the Day

Incorporating a new word into your daily routine can help build your vocabulary. Use the word in sentences throughout the day to reinforce your learning.

Example:

- Word of the Day: "Serendipity"
- Sentence: "It was sheer serendipity that we met at the café."

Practice Exercise:

Try replacing the underlined words with more vivid or precise vocabulary:

1. The sunset was very beautiful.
2. She was very tired after the long day.
3. His speech was very interesting.

Practice Exercise:

Create sentences using each of the following words. Pay attention to their meanings and use them correctly in context:

1. Magnificent
2. Tedious
3. Jubilant
4. Ominous
5. Elated

Using Context Clues for Meaning

Context clues are hints within a sentence or paragraph that help define unfamiliar words. By learning to use context clues, you can improve your reading comprehension and expand your vocabulary.

Types of Context Clues

1. **Definition Clues:** The word's meaning is explained in the sentence.
   - "Archaeology, the study of ancient cultures, is a fascinating field."

2. **Synonym Clues:** A synonym or similar word is used.
   - "The artist's latest work is a masterpiece, a true magnum opus."

3. **Antonym Clues:** An antonym or opposite word is used to define the unfamiliar word.
   - "Unlike his boisterous brother, he is quite reticent."

4. **Inference Clues:** The meaning is not directly stated but can be inferred from the context.
   - "She felt a pang of nostalgia as she walked through her old neighborhood, reminiscing about the past."

Practice Exercise:

Determine the meaning of the underlined words using context clues:

1. The **effervescent** soda fizzed over the top of the glass.

2. His **parsimonious** nature was evident when he refused to buy new clothes.

3. The **cacophony** of the city streets was overwhelming to the newcomers.

Practice Exercise:

Write a short paragraph using the following words. Provide enough context clues to help a reader understand the meanings of the words:

1. Ambivalent

2. Melancholy

3. Exuberant

4. Indispensable

5. Luminous

Recognizing and Correcting Common Errors

Common grammatical errors can undermine the clarity and professionalism of your writing. By learning to recognize and correct these errors, you can significantly improve your writing quality.

Subject-Verb Agreement

Ensure that subjects and verbs agree in number. Singular subjects take singular verbs, and plural subjects take plural verbs.

Example:

- Incorrect: "The list of items are long."

- Correct: "The list of items is long."

Pronoun-Antecedent Agreement

Pronouns must agree with their antecedents in number and gender.

Example:

- Incorrect: "Each student must submit their homework."

- Correct: "Each student must submit his or her homework."

Misplaced Modifiers

Modifiers should be placed next to the word they are meant to describe.

Example:

- Incorrect: "She almost drove her kids to school every day."
- Correct: "She drove her kids to school almost every day."

Practice Exercise:

Correct the following sentences:

1. The committee are planning a big event.
2. Everyone must bring their own lunch.
3. She served cake to the children on paper plates.

Practice Exercise:

Identify and correct the errors in these sentences:

1. Neither of the boys have completed their homework.
2. The bouquet of roses were beautiful.
3. Anyone can bring their friend to the party.
4. She almost spent all her savings on the vacation.
5. The team are practicing for their next game.

Understanding Idioms and Phrases

Idioms and phrases add color and character to the language. Understanding their meanings and how to use them correctly can enhance your writing.

Common Idioms

1. **Break the ice:** To initiate conversation in a social setting.
   - "At the party, she told a joke to break the ice."

2. **Hit the nail on the head:** To be exactly right about something.
   - "Her analysis of the problem hit the nail on the head."

3. **Under the weather:** Feeling ill.
   - "He couldn't come to work because he was feeling under the weather."

Practice Exercise:

Use the following idioms in sentences:

1. Spill the beans
2. Piece of cake
3. Bite the bullet

Practice Exercise:

Rewrite the following sentences using idioms from the list provided:

1. It was very easy for her to pass the test.
2. He finally revealed the secret.
3. She decided to face the difficult situation bravely.

Practice Exercise:

Explain the meanings of these idioms and use each in a sentence:

1. A blessing in disguise
2. Burn the midnight oil
3. Let the cat out of the bag
4. Through thick and thin
5. On cloud nine

Sentence Variety and Style

Varying sentence structure and style can make your writing more interesting and dynamic. Mixing different types of sentences keeps the reader engaged and helps to emphasize different points.

Combining Sentences

Combine simple sentences to form compound or complex sentences for variety and depth.

Example:

- Simple: "The sun set. The sky turned orange."
- Combined: "The sun set, and the sky turned orange."

Using Different Sentence Types

1. **Simple Sentence:** A single independent clause.
   - "She enjoys reading."
2. **Compound Sentence:** Two independent clauses joined by a conjunction.
   - "She enjoys reading, and she also likes painting."
3. **Complex Sentence:** An independent clause joined by one or more dependent clauses.
   - "Although she enjoys reading, she finds little time for it."
4. **Compound-Complex Sentence:** At least two independent clauses and one or more dependent clauses.
   - "She enjoys reading, but because she is so busy, she often reads only before bed."

Practice Exercise:

Rewrite the following sentences to add variety:

1. The dog barked. The mailman ran away.
2. She was tired. She went to bed early.
3. It was raining. We decided to stay indoors.

Practice Exercise:

Identify the sentence type (simple, compound, complex, or compound-complex) and rewrite it using a different structure:

1. She reads every day.
2. He wanted to go to the park, but it was too late.
3. When the bell rang, the students quickly left the classroom.
4. She loves to cook, and she often tries new recipes because she enjoys it.

Application in Context

To bring it all together, let's apply these rules in context. Consider the following paragraph and the steps taken to enhance it:

Original Paragraph:

"The project was challenging. We had a lot of problems. The team worked hard. Finally, we completed it successfully."

Enhanced Paragraph:

"Despite the project's challenging nature, we encountered numerous problems along the way. However, the team's diligent efforts paid off, and we successfully completed the project."

Steps Taken:

1. **Combine Sentences:** Merged simple sentences into compound and complex sentences.
2. **Enhanced Vocabulary:** Replaced generic words with more specific ones (e.g., 'challenging nature' instead of 'challenging').
3. **Added Detail:** Included more information to provide context and clarity.

Practice Exercise:

Revise the following paragraph to improve sentence variety, vocabulary, and clarity:

"We went to the park. It was a sunny day. We had a picnic. The children played games. Everyone had a good time."

Practice Exercise:

Edit the following paragraph to correct grammar errors, enhance word choice, and improve sentence structure:

"She loves to travel. She has been to many countries. Her favorite place is Italy. The food is great. The scenery is beautiful. She plans to visit again next year."

Additional Grammar Rules and Examples

To further your understanding, let's explore more advanced grammar rules along with examples to illustrate their proper usage.

Parallel Structure

Parallel structure, or parallelism, means using the same pattern of words to show that two or more ideas have the same level of importance. This can happen at the word, phrase, or clause level.

Example:

- Incorrect: "She likes to jog, running, and to swim."

- Correct: "She likes jogging, running, and swimming."

Consistent Verb Tense

Maintain the same verb tense within a sentence or paragraph to avoid confusion.

Example:

- Incorrect: "She was reading when her phone rings."

- Correct: "She was reading when her phone rang."

Active vs. Passive Voice

Active voice makes sentences clearer and more direct. In active voice, the subject performs the action. In passive voice, the action is performed on the subject.

Example:

- Active: "The chef cooked a delicious meal."

- Passive: "A delicious meal was cooked by the chef."

Relative Clauses

Relative clauses provide extra information about a noun. They begin with relative pronouns like 'who', 'whom', 'whose', 'which', or 'that'.

Example:

- "The book, which was on the table, is missing."

- "The person who called you is my friend."

Subjective vs. Objective Pronouns

Use subjective pronouns (I, you, he, she, it, we, they) as subjects and objective pronouns (me, you, him, her, it, us, them) as objects.

Example:

- Subjective: "She and I went to the market."

- Objective: "The gift is for him and me."

Possessive Pronouns

Possessive pronouns show ownership and include words like my, your, his, her, its, our, their.

Example:

- "This is my book."

- "Their house is beautiful."

Comparatives and Superlatives

Comparatives compare two things, usually ending in '-er' or using 'more'. Superlatives compare three or more things, usually ending in '-est' or using 'most'.

Example:

- Comparative: "She is taller than her brother."
- Superlative: "She is the tallest person in her family."

Double Negatives

Avoid using double negatives, which can create confusion and imply the opposite of what you mean.

Example:

- Incorrect: "I don't need no help."
- Correct: "I don't need any help."

Countable vs. Uncountable Nouns

Countable nouns can be counted (e.g., one apple, two apples), while uncountable nouns cannot be counted (e.g., water, rice).

Example:

- Countable: "There are three books on the table."
- Uncountable: "There is some water in the glass."

Articles

Use 'a' and 'an' for non-specific items, and 'the' for specific items.

Example:

- "I saw a cat." (any cat)
- "I saw the cat." (a specific cat)

Prepositional Phrases

A prepositional phrase starts with a preposition and ends with a noun or pronoun. It provides additional details about the action.

Example:

- "The book on the table is mine."
- "She walked through the park."

Pronoun-Antecedent Agreement

Ensure that pronouns agree with their antecedents in number and gender.

Example:

- Incorrect: "Each student must bring their own pencil."
- Correct: "Each student must bring his or her own pencil."

Direct and Indirect Objects

A direct object receives the action of the verb, while an indirect object is the recipient of the direct object.

Example:

- Direct Object: "She wrote a letter."
- Indirect Object: "She wrote her friend a letter."

Gerunds and Infinitives

A gerund is a verb ending in '-ing' that functions as a noun, while an infinitive is the base form of a verb preceded by 'to'.

Example:

- Gerund: "Swimming is fun."
- Infinitive: "To swim is fun."

Sentence Fragments

Avoid sentence fragments by ensuring each sentence has a subject and a verb and expresses a complete thought.

Example:

- Fragment: "Because I was tired."
- Complete Sentence: "Because I was tired, I went to bed early."

Run-On Sentences

Run-on sentences occur when two or more independent clauses are joined without proper punctuation or conjunctions.

Example:

- Incorrect: "I love to write it is my favorite hobby."
- Correct: "I love to write; it is my favorite hobby."

More Examples and Exercises

Exercise 1: Parallel Structure Practice

Identify and correct the parallel structure errors in the following sentences:

1. "She likes to jog, running, and to swim."
   - Corrected: "She likes jogging, running, and swimming."
2. "The manager asked for the report to be concise, accurate, and written with clarity."
   - Corrected: "The manager asked for the report to be concise, accurate, and clear."

Exercise 2: Verb Tense Consistency

Ensure consistent verb tense in the following sentences:

1. "She was singing when he comes in."
   - Corrected: "She was singing when he came in."
2. "They finished their project and then they go to the party."
   - Corrected: "They finished their project and then they went to the party."

Exercise 3: Active vs. Passive Voice

Rewrite the following sentences in active voice:

1. "The cake was eaten by the children."
   - Active: "The children ate the cake."
2. "A new policy was implemented by the company."
   - Active: "The company implemented a new policy."

Exercise 4: Relative Clauses

Combine the sentences using relative clauses:

1. "The book is on the table. It is mine."
   - Combined: "The book that is on the table is mine."
2. "The woman called you. She is my friend."
   - Combined: "The woman who called you is my friend."

Exercise 5: Countable and Uncountable Nouns

Identify whether the following nouns are countable or uncountable:

1. "Milk" - Uncountable
2. "Car" - Countable
3. "Information" - Uncountable
4. "Apple" - Countable

Application in Context

To bring it all together, let's apply these rules in context. Consider the following paragraph and the steps taken to enhance it:

Original Paragraph:

"The project was challenging. We had a lot of problems. The team worked hard. Finally, we completed it successfully."

Enhanced Paragraph:

"Despite the project's challenging nature, we encountered numerous problems along the way. However, the team's diligent efforts paid off, and we successfully completed the project."

Steps Taken:

1. **Combine Sentences:** Merged simple sentences into compound and complex sentences.

2. **Enhanced Vocabulary:** Replaced generic words with more specific ones (e.g., 'challenging nature' instead of 'challenging').

3. **Added Detail:** Included more information to provide context and clarity.

Practice Exercise:

Revise the following paragraph to improve sentence variety, vocabulary, and clarity:

"We went to the park. It was a sunny day. We had a picnic. The children played games. Everyone had a good time."

Improved Paragraph:

"On a sunny day, we decided to visit the park. We enjoyed a delightful picnic while the children played various games. Overall, it was a fun and relaxing outing for everyone."

Practice Exercise:

Edit the following paragraph to correct grammar errors, enhance word choice, and improve sentence structure:

"She loves to travel. She has been to many countries. Her favorite place is Italy. The food is great. The scenery is beautiful. She plans to visit again next year."

Improved Paragraph:

"She has a passion for travel and has visited many countries. Her favorite destination is Italy, known for its delicious cuisine and breathtaking scenery. She plans to return there next year to explore even more."

Additional Grammar Rules and Examples

To further your understanding, let's explore more advanced grammar rules along with examples to illustrate their proper usage.

Parallel Structure

Parallel structure, or parallelism, means using the same pattern of words to show that two or more ideas have the same level of importance. This can happen at the word, phrase, or clause level.

Example:

- Incorrect: "She likes to jog, running, and to swim."

- Correct: "She likes jogging, running, and swimming."

Consistent Verb Tense

Maintain the same verb tense within a sentence or paragraph to avoid confusion.

Example:

- Incorrect: "She was reading when her phone rings."

- Correct: "She was reading when her phone rang."

Active vs. Passive Voice

Active voice makes sentences clearer and more direct. In active voice, the subject performs the action. In passive voice, the action is performed on the subject.

Example:

- Active: "The chef cooked a delicious meal."
- Passive: "A delicious meal was cooked by the chef."

Relative Clauses

Relative clauses provide extra information about a noun. They begin with relative pronouns like 'who', 'whom', 'whose', 'which', or 'that'.

Example:

- "The book, which was on the table, is missing."
- "The person who called you is my friend."

Subjective vs. Objective Pronouns

Use subjective pronouns (I, you, he, she, it, we, they) as subjects and objective pronouns (me, you, him, her, it, us, them) as objects.

Example:

- Subjective: "She and I went to the market."
- Objective: "The gift is for him and me."

Possessive Pronouns

Possessive pronouns show ownership and include words like my, your, his, her, its, our, their.

Example:

- "This is my book."
- "Their house is beautiful."

Comparatives and Superlatives

Comparatives compare two things, usually ending in '-er' or using 'more'. Superlatives compare three or more things, usually ending in '-est' or using 'most'.

Example:

- Comparative: "She is taller than her brother."
- Superlative: "She is the tallest person in her family."

Double Negatives

Avoid using double negatives, which can create confusion and imply the opposite of what you mean.

Example:

- Incorrect: "I don't need no help."
- Correct: "I don't need any help."

Countable vs. Uncountable Nouns

Countable nouns can be counted (e.g., one apple, two apples), while uncountable nouns cannot be counted (e.g., water, rice).

Example:

- Countable: "There are three books on the table."
- Uncountable: "There is some water in the glass."

Articles

Use 'a' and 'an' for non-specific items, and 'the' for specific items.

Example:

- "I saw a cat." (any cat)
- "I saw the cat." (a specific cat)

Prepositional Phrases

A prepositional phrase starts with a preposition and ends with a noun or pronoun. It provides additional details about the action.

Example:

- "The book on the table is mine."
- "She walked through the park."

Pronoun-Antecedent Agreement

Ensure that pronouns agree with their antecedents in number and gender.

A direct object receives the action of the verb, while an indirect object is the recipient of the direct object.

Example:

- Direct Object: "She wrote a letter."
- Indirect Object: "She wrote her friend a letter."

Gerunds and Infinitives

A gerund is a verb ending in '-ing' that functions as a noun, while an infinitive is the base form of a verb preceded by 'to'.

Example:

- Gerund: "Swimming is fun."
- Infinitive: "To swim is fun."

Sentence Fragments

More Examples and Exercises

Exercise 1: Parallel Structure Practice

Identify and correct the parallel structure errors in the following sentences:

1. "She likes to jog, running, and to swim."
   - Corrected: "She likes jogging, running, and swimming."

2. "The manager asked for the report to be concise, accurate, and written with clarity."

Example:

- Incorrect: "Each student must bring their own pencil."
- Correct: "Each student must bring his or her own pencil."

Direct and Indirect Objects

Avoid sentence fragments by ensuring each sentence has a subject and a verb and expresses a complete thought.

Example:

- Fragment: "Because I was tired."
- Complete Sentence: "Because I was tired, I went to bed early."

Run-On Sentences

Run-on sentences occur when two or more independent clauses are joined without proper punctuation or conjunctions.

Example:

- Incorrect: "I love to write it is my favorite hobby."
- Correct: "I love to write; it is my favorite hobby."

   - Corrected: "The manager asked for the report to be concise, accurate, and clear."

Exercise 2: Verb Tense Consistency

Ensure consistent verb tense in the following sentences:

1. "She was singing when he comes in."
   - Corrected: "She was singing when he came in."

2. "They finished their project and then they go to the party."

- Corrected: "They finished their project and then they went to the party."

Exercise 3: Active vs. Passive Voice

Rewrite the following sentences in active voice:

1. "The cake was eaten by the children."
   - Active: "The children ate the cake."
2. "A new policy was implemented by the company."
   - Active: "The company implemented a new policy."

Exercise 4: Relative Clauses

Combine the sentences using relative clauses:

1. "The book is on the table. It is mine."
   - Combined: "The book that is on the table is mine."
2. "The woman called you. She is my friend."
   - Combined: "The woman who called you is my friend."

Exercise 5: Countable and Uncountable Nouns

Identify whether the following nouns are countable or uncountable:

1. "Milk" - Uncountable
2. "Car" - Countable
3. "Information" - Uncountable
4. "Apple" - Countable

Application in Context

To bring it all together, let's apply these rules in context. Consider the following paragraph and the steps taken to enhance it:

Original Paragraph:

"The project was challenging. We had a lot of problems. The team worked hard. Finally, we completed it successfully."

Enhanced Paragraph:

"Despite the project's challenging nature, we encountered numerous problems along the way. However, the team's diligent efforts paid off, and we successfully completed the project."

Steps Taken:

1. **Combine Sentences:** Merged simple sentences into compound and complex sentences.
2. **Enhanced Vocabulary:** Replaced generic words with more specific ones (e.g., 'challenging nature' instead of 'challenging').
3. **Added Detail:** Included more information to provide context and clarity.

Practice Exercise:

Revise the following paragraph to improve sentence variety, vocabulary, and clarity:

"We went to the park. It was a sunny day. We had a picnic. The children played games. Everyone had a good time."

Improved Paragraph:

"On a sunny day, we decided to visit the park. We enjoyed a delightful picnic while the children played various games. Overall, it was a fun and relaxing outing for everyone."

Practice Exercise:

Edit the following paragraph to correct grammar errors, enhance word choice, and improve sentence structure:

"She loves to travel. She has been to many countries. Her favorite place is Italy. The food is great. The scenery is beautiful. She plans to visit again next year."

Improved Paragraph:

"She has a passion for travel and has visited many countries. Her favorite destination is Italy, known for its delicious cuisine and breathtaking scenery. She plans to return there next year to explore even more."

Additional Grammar Rules and Examples

To further your understanding, let's explore more advanced grammar rules along with examples to illustrate their proper usage.

Parallel Structure

Parallel structure, or parallelism, means using the same pattern of words to show that two or more ideas have the same level of importance. This can happen at the word, phrase, or clause level.

Example:

- Incorrect: "She likes to jog, running, and to swim."
- Correct: "She likes jogging, running, and swimming."

Consistent Verb Tense

Maintain the same verb tense within a sentence or paragraph to avoid confusion.

Example:

- Incorrect: "She was reading when her phone rings."
- Correct: "She was reading when her phone rang."

Active vs. Passive Voice

Active voice makes sentences clearer and more direct. In active voice, the subject performs the action. In passive voice, the action is performed on the subject.

Example:

- Active: "The chef cooked a delicious meal."
- Passive: "A delicious meal was cooked by the chef."

Relative Clauses

Relative clauses provide extra information about a noun. They begin with relative pronouns like 'who', 'whom', 'whose', 'which', or 'that'.

Example:

- "The book, which was on the table, is missing."
- "The person who called you is my friend."

Subjective vs. Objective Pronouns

Use subjective pronouns (I, you, he, she, it, we, they) as subjects and objective pronouns (me, you, him, her, it, us, them) as objects.

Example:

- Subjective: "She and I went to the market."
- Objective: "The gift is for him and me."

Possessive Pronouns

Possessive pronouns show ownership and include words like my, your, his, her, its, our, their.

Example:

- "This is my book."
- "Their house is beautiful."

Comparatives and Superlatives

Comparatives compare two things, usually ending in '-er' or using 'more'. Superlatives compare three or more things, usually ending in '-est' or using 'most'.

Example:

- Comparative: "She is taller than her brother."

- Superlative: "She is the tallest person in her family."

Double Negatives

Avoid using double negatives, which can create confusion and imply the opposite of what you mean.

Example:

- Incorrect: "I don't need no help."

- Correct: "I don't need any help."

Countable vs. Uncountable Nouns

Countable nouns can be counted (e.g., one apple, two apples), while uncountable nouns cannot be counted (e.g., water, rice).

Example:

- Countable: "There are three books on the table."

- Uncountable: "There is some water in the glass."

Articles

Use 'a' and 'an' for non-specific items, and 'the' for specific items.

Example:

- "I saw a cat." (any cat)

- "I saw the cat." (a specific cat)

Prepositional Phrases

A prepositional phrase starts with a preposition and ends with a noun or pronoun. It provides additional details about the action.

Example:

- "The book on the table is mine."

- "She walked through the park."

Pronoun-Antecedent Agreement

Ensure that pronouns agree with their antecedents in number and gender.

Example:

- Incorrect: "Each student must bring their own pencil."

- Correct: "Each student must bring his or her own pencil."

Direct and Indirect Objects

A direct object receives the action of the verb, while an indirect object is the recipient of the direct object.

Example:

- Direct Object: "She wrote a letter."

- Indirect Object: "She wrote her friend a letter."

Gerunds and Infinitives

A gerund is a verb ending in '-ing' that functions as a noun, while an infinitive is the base form of a verb preceded by 'to'.

Example:

- Gerund: "Swimming is fun."

- Infinitive: "To swim is fun."

Sentence Fragments

Avoid sentence fragments by ensuring each sentence has a subject and a verb and expresses a complete thought.

Example:

- Fragment: "Because I was tired."

- Complete Sentence: "Because I was tired, I went to bed early."

Run-On Sentences

Run-on sentences occur when two or more independent clauses are joined without proper punctuation or conjunctions.

Example:

- Incorrect: "I love to write it is my favorite hobby."
- Correct: "I love to write; it is my favorite hobby."

More Examples and Exercises

Exercise 1: Parallel Structure Practice

Identify and correct the parallel structure errors in the following sentences:

1. "She likes to jog, running, and to swim."
   - Corrected: "She likes jogging, running, and swimming."
2. "The manager asked for the report to be concise, accurate, and written with clarity."
   - Corrected: "The manager asked for the report to be concise, accurate, and clear."

Exercise 2: Verb Tense Consistency

Ensure consistent verb tense in the following sentences:

1. "She was singing when he comes in."
   - Corrected: "She was singing when he came in."
2. "They finished their project and then they go to the party."
   - Corrected: "They finished their project and then they went to the party."

Exercise 3: Active vs. Passive Voice

Rewrite the following sentences in active voice:

1. "The cake was eaten by the children."
   - Active: "The children ate the cake."
2. "A new policy was implemented by the company."
   - Active: "The company implemented a new policy."

Exercise 4: Relative Clauses

Combine the sentences using relative clauses:

1. "The book is on the table. It is mine."
   - Combined: "The book that is on the table is mine."
2. "The woman called you. She is my friend."
   - Combined: "The woman who called you is my friend."

Exercise 5: Countable and Uncountable Nouns

Identify whether the following nouns are countable or uncountable:

1. "Milk" - Uncountable
2. "Car" - Countable
3. "Information" - Uncountable
4. "Apple" - Countable

Application in Context

To bring it all together, let's apply these rules in context. Consider the following paragraph and the steps taken to enhance it:

Original Paragraph:

"The project was challenging. We had a lot of problems. The team worked hard. Finally, we completed it successfully."

Enhanced Paragraph:

"Despite the project's challenging nature, we encountered numerous problems along the way. However, the team's diligent efforts paid off, and we successfully completed the project."

Steps Taken:

1. **Combine Sentences:** Merged simple sentences into compound and complex sentences.

2. **Enhanced Vocabulary:** Replaced generic words with more specific ones (e.g., 'challenging nature' instead of 'challenging').

3. **Added Detail:** Included more information to provide context and clarity.

Practice Exercise:

Revise the following paragraph to improve sentence variety, vocabulary, and clarity:

"We went to the park. It was a sunny day. We had a picnic. The children played games. Everyone had a good time."

Improved Paragraph:

"On a sunny day, we decided to visit the park. We enjoyed a delightful picnic while the children played various games. Overall, it was a fun and relaxing outing for everyone."

Practice Exercise:

Edit the following paragraph to correct grammar errors, enhance word choice, and improve sentence structure:

"She loves to travel. She has been to many countries. Her favorite place is Italy. The food is great. The scenery is beautiful. She plans to visit again next year."

Improved Paragraph:

"She has a passion for travel and has visited many countries. Her favorite destination is Italy, known for its delicious cuisine and breathtaking scenery. She plans to return there next year to explore even more."

Further Applications and Practice

Contextual Editing

Take the following passage and edit it for grammatical accuracy, clarity, and style:

Original Passage:

"John and his friend were walking down the street. They were going to the new café that opened last week. John didn't like the coffee, but his friend said it was okay. They talked about their plans for the weekend. John wanted to go hiking, but his friend preferred to stay home and watch movies."

Edited Passage:

"John and his friend strolled down the street toward the newly opened café. While John found the coffee disappointing, his friend thought it was acceptable. They discussed their weekend plans; John was eager to go hiking, whereas his friend preferred to stay home and watch movies."

Analysis and Steps Taken:

1. **Word Choice:** Replaced "were walking" with "strolled" for more vivid imagery.

2. **Sentence Variety:** Combined sentences to create compound and complex structures.

3. **Clarity and Style:** Added specific details and transitions to enhance the flow and clarity of the passage.

Practical Exercise:

Edit the following passage to improve grammar, clarity, and style:

"Maria went to the market. She bought fruits, vegetables, and bread. The market was crowded. She saw her friend there. They talked for a while. Then Maria went home. She made a salad for lunch. It was delicious."

Extended Practice:

Edit the following longer passage, focusing on grammar, vocabulary, sentence variety, and overall clarity:

"Thomas decided to visit the museum on his day off. He had heard about a new exhibit on ancient civilizations. When he arrived, he bought a ticket and went inside. The exhibit was very interesting. He learned a lot about the history and culture of different ancient civilizations. After spending several hours at the museum, he felt hungry and decided to have lunch at a nearby restaurant. The food was good. After lunch, he took a walk in the park. It was a relaxing way to end his day."

Extended Edited Passage:

"On his day off, Thomas chose to visit the museum to see a new exhibit on ancient civilizations. Upon arrival, he purchased a ticket and entered the museum. The exhibit was fascinating, offering a wealth of information about the history and culture of various ancient civilizations. After several hours of exploration, Thomas felt hungry and opted for lunch at a nearby restaurant, where the food was delightful. Following lunch, he enjoyed a leisurely walk in the park, providing a relaxing conclusion to his day."

Steps Taken:

1. **Enhanced Vocabulary:** Replaced generic words with more descriptive alternatives (e.g., "chose" instead of "decided").

2. **Sentence Variety:** Combined and restructured sentences to create a more engaging narrative.

3. **Clarity and Flow:** Added transitions and specific details to improve readability and coherence.

By practicing these techniques regularly, you can develop a stronger command of grammar and enhance your writing style. Remember, consistent practice and application of these principles are key to becoming a proficient and confident writer.

CONCLUSION
READING STRATEGIES FOR SUCCESS

The ATI TEAS (Test of Essential Academic Skills) is a vital exam for those pursuing a career in nursing. It evaluates your abilities in four key areas: Reading, Mathematics, Science, and English and Language Usage. Excelling in the TEAS requires a combination of knowledge and strategic test-taking skills. This chapter offers practical tips to help you tackle the exam effectively.

Preparing for the Test

1. **Understand the Test Format**: The TEAS is divided into four sections with multiple-choice questions. Familiarize yourself with the format and types of questions you will encounter. This knowledge will help you navigate the test more confidently.

2. **Practice Under Timed Conditions**: Take practice tests under timed conditions to simulate the actual exam environment. This will help you get used to the pace of the test and improve your time management skills.

3. **Review Key Concepts**: Focus on areas where you feel less confident. Use study guides, flashcards, and practice questions to reinforce your knowledge. Consistent review can significantly boost your confidence and performance.

During the Test

1. Managing Your Time

- **Pace Yourself**: Each section of the TEAS has a specific time limit. Divide your time per question and try to stick to it. If a question is taking too long, mark it and move on. You can return to it later if you have time.

- **Monitor the Clock**: Keep an eye on the clock without obsessing over it. Periodically check the time to ensure you are on track to complete each section.

2. Reading Questions Carefully

- **Understand the Question**: Read each question thoroughly to ensure you understand what is being asked. Misinterpreting a question can lead to incorrect answers even if you know the correct information.

- **Look for Key Words**: Pay attention to key words such as "not," "except," "best," and "most." These words can change the meaning of the question and the correct answer.

3. Answering Strategies

- **Answer Easy Questions First**: Start with questions you find easy. This builds confidence and secures quick points. It also leaves you more time to tackle difficult questions later.

- **Eliminate Wrong Answers**: Use the process of elimination to narrow down your choices. Even if you are unsure of the correct answer, eliminating obviously incorrect options increases your chances of guessing correctly.

- **Trust Your Instincts**: Often, your first instinct is correct. Avoid second-guessing yourself unless you find clear evidence that another answer is correct.

- **Move On and Return**: If a question is taking too long, mark it and move on. Return to it later if time permits. This ensures you do not get stuck and run out of time.

4. Staying Calm and Focused

- **Stay Relaxed**: Anxiety can hinder your performance. Take deep breaths and stay calm. A positive mindset can make a significant difference in how you perform.

- **Take Short Breaks**: If the test format allows, take brief breaks to rest your mind. Stand up, stretch, and take deep breaths to refocus your energy.

- **Block Out Distractions**: Concentrate solely on the test. Ignore distractions around you and keep your attention on the task at hand.

5. Reviewing Your Answers

- **Use Remaining Time Wisely**: If you finish a section early, use the remaining time to review your answers. Look for any mistakes or questions you may have skipped.

- **Check for Obvious Errors**: Ensure you have not misread questions or marked the wrong answers. Correct any errors you find.

Section-Specific Tips

- **Reading**: Skim the passages to get a general idea before diving into the questions. Focus on the main ideas and supporting details.

- **Mathematics**: Write down your calculations to avoid mistakes. Use estimation to quickly eliminate unreasonable answer choices.

- **Science**: Focus on understanding concepts rather than memorizing facts. Apply your knowledge to interpret data and answer questions.

- **English and Language Usage**: Pay attention to grammar, punctuation, and sentence structure. Review basic grammar rules to ensure accuracy.

VIDEO

FOR THE VIDEO COURSE SCAN THIS QR CODE

OR

CLICK HERE

BONUSES

FOR ATI TEAS TEST FLASHCARDS & PRACTICE TESTS SCAN THIS QR CODE

OR

CLICK HERE

THE LAST STEP IS YOU!

Remember that you've already come a long way.

Your dedication to studying and mastering the material has equipped you with the knowledge you need.

Now, the final step is to believe in yourself.

Embrace the confidence that comes from knowing you've done your best to prepare. Trust in your abilities and the hard work you've put in.

The TEAS is just one step on your journey to a rewarding career in nursing, and you have the power to succeed.

Stay calm, stay focused, and remember to breathe. Each question is an opportunity to showcase what you know. If you encounter a challenging question, take a deep breath and use the strategies you've learned to tackle it.

Believe in your potential, trust in your preparation, and know that you are capable of achieving your goals.

You've got this!

Good luck!

Made in the USA
Columbia, SC
16 April 2025

56744607R00078